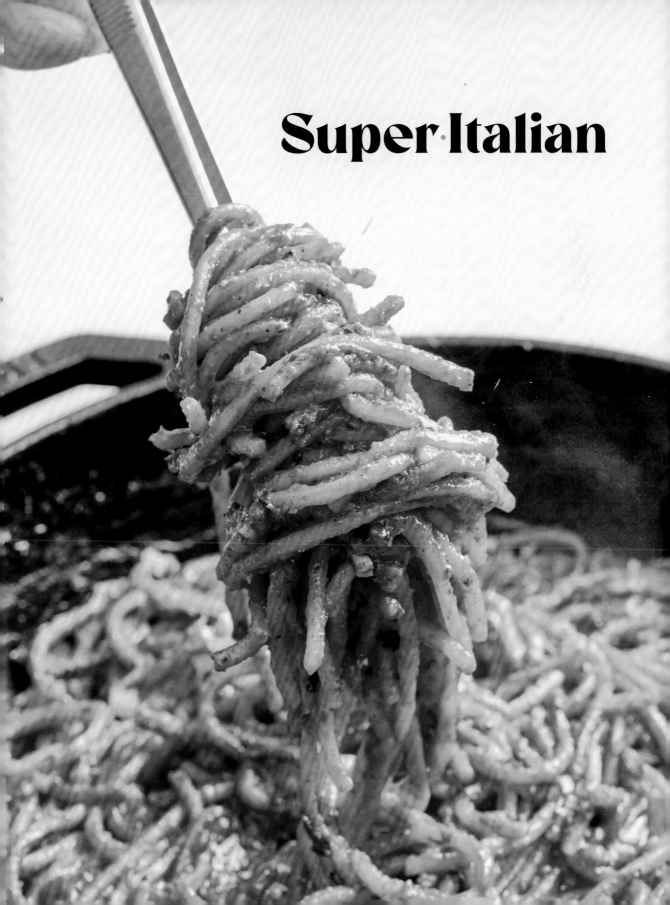

Super·Italian

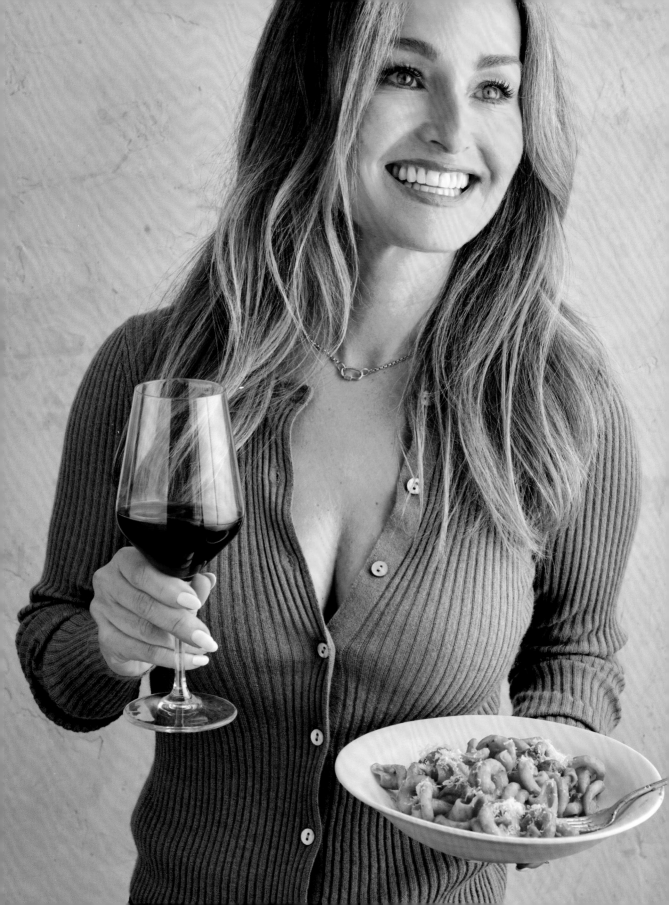

Super·Italian

More Than 110 Indulgent Recipes Using Italy's Healthiest Foods

Giada De Laurentiis

RODALE

NEW YORK

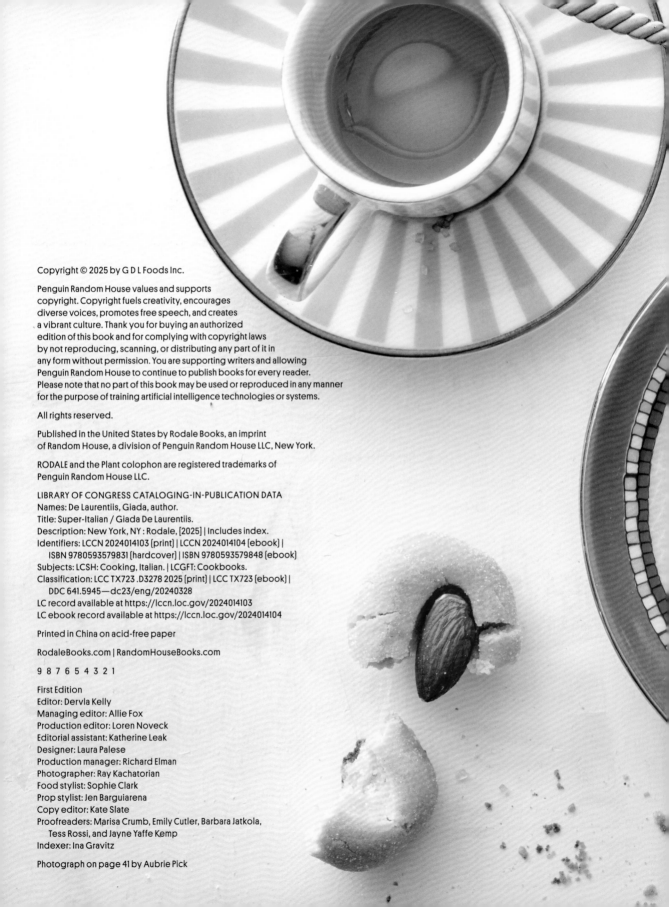

Published in the United States by Rodale Books, an imprint
of Random House, a division of Penguin Random House LLC, New York.

RODALE and the Plant colophon are registered trademarks of
Penguin Random House LLC.

LIBRARY OF CONGRESS CATALOGING-IN-PUBLICATION DATA
Names: De Laurentiis, Giada, author.
Title: Super-Italian / Giada De Laurentiis.
Description: New York, NY : Rodale, [2025] | Includes index.
Identifiers: LCCN 2024014103 [print] | LCCN 2024014104 [ebook] |
    ISBN 9780593579831 [hardcover] | ISBN 9780593579848 [ebook]
Subjects: LCSH: Cooking, Italian. | LCGFT: Cookbooks.
Classification: LCC TX723 .D3278 2025 [print] | LCC TX723 [ebook] |
    DDC 641.5945—dc23/eng/20240328
LC record available at https://lccn.loc.gov/2024014103
LC ebook record available at https://lccn.loc.gov/2024014104

Printed in China on acid-free paper

RodaleBooks.com | RandomHouseBooks.com

9 8 7 6 5 4 3 2 1

First Edition
Editor: Dervla Kelly
Managing editor: Allie Fox
Production editor: Loren Noveck
Editorial assistant: Katherine Leak
Designer: Laura Palese
Production manager: Richard Elman
Photographer: Ray Kachatorian
Food stylist: Sophie Clark
Prop stylist: Jen Barguiarena
Copy editor: Kate Slate
Proofreaders: Marisa Crumb, Emily Cutler, Barbara Jatkola,
    Tess Rossi, and Jayne Yaffe Kemp
Indexer: Ina Gravitz

Photograph on page 41 by Aubrie Pick

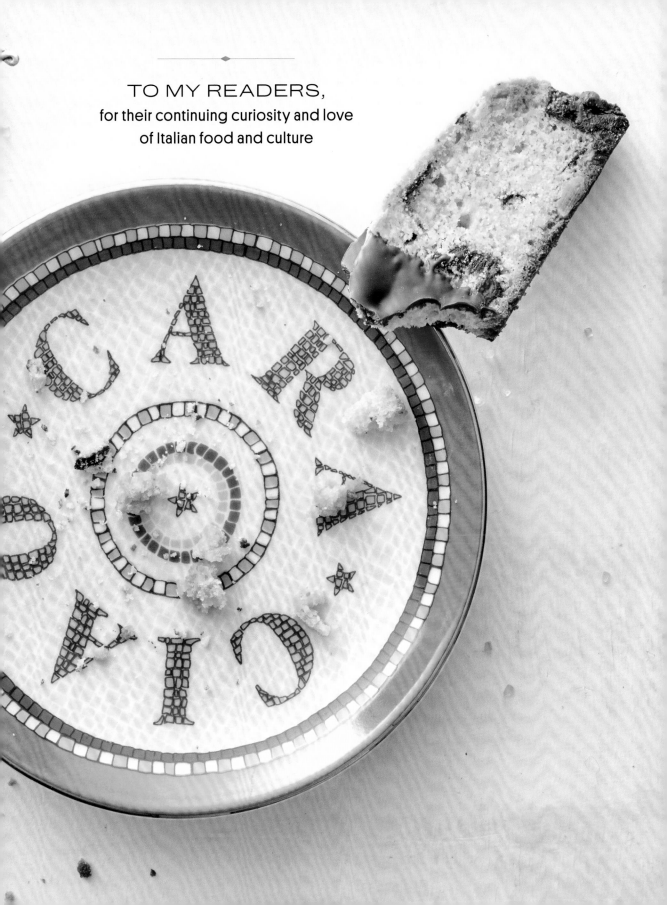

TO MY READERS,
for their continuing curiosity and love
of Italian food and culture

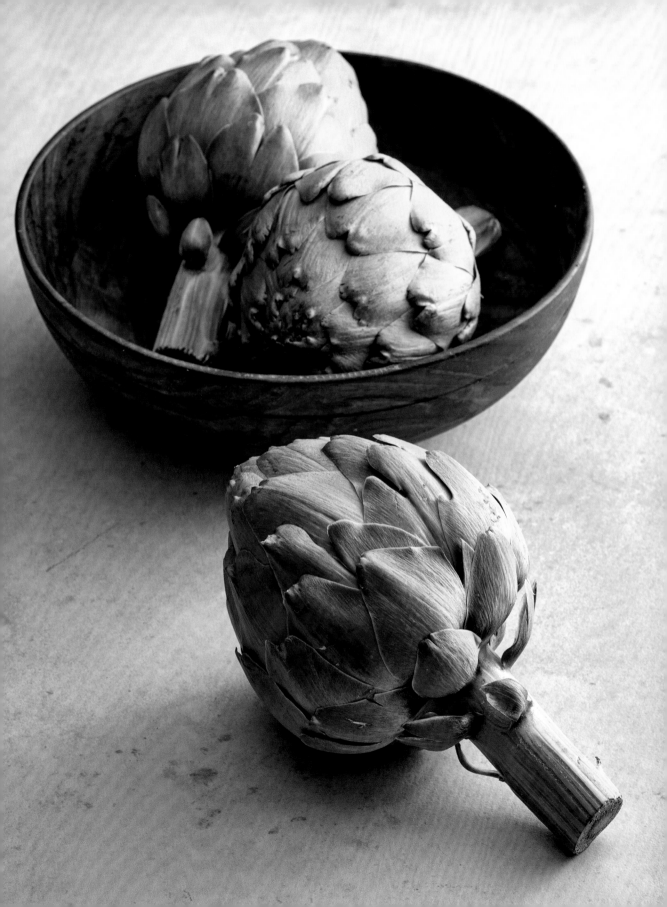

Contents

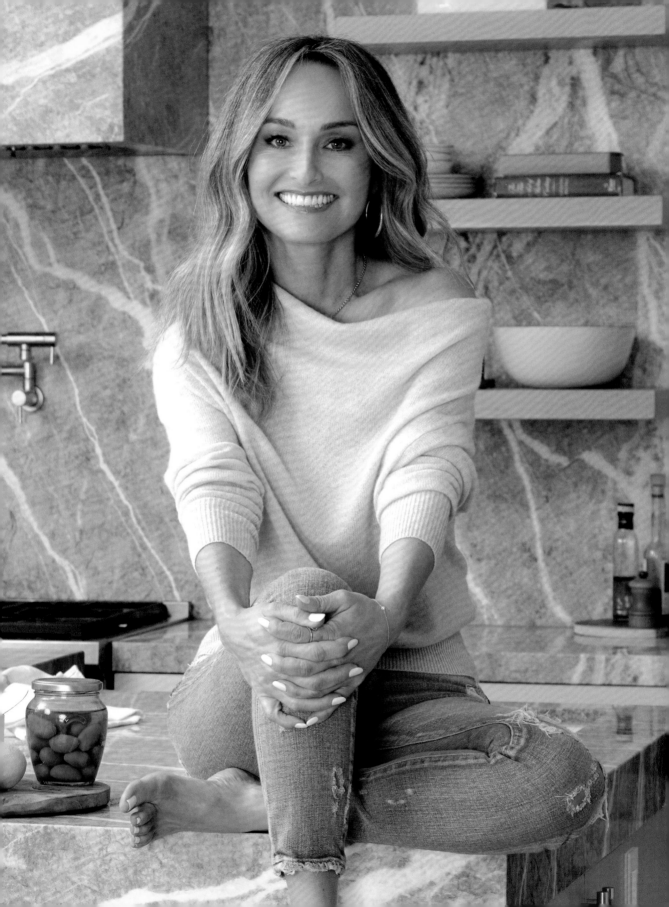

Introduction

IF THE PAST FEW years have taught us anything, it's that life involves a series of pivots. Certainly, that has been true for me and my journey through the world of food and cooking.

I knew from a very young age that I wanted to be involved in the food world in some capacity, although it took me a while to articulate it— even to myself. When I was a kid, new to this country and feeling a bit like a fish out of water, mealtimes with my extended family were the best time of the day, and when we weren't eating we were talking about food and thinking about what we'd eat later. That might seem a bit extreme, but I didn't know any different. I thought everyone cooked with their grandparents, and loved food the way my family did.

In my teen years, I haunted the aisles of my grandfather's incredible gourmet food destination, DDL Foodshow, where patrons could buy everything from prepared foods to pastries, pizzas to pignolis. Working there after school, seeing how excited people were by the ingredients my grandfather imported to the United States, many of which were not available elsewhere in this country, instilled a huge

respect in me for the power of food, specifically Italian food, to enrich people's lives. I knew then that I wanted to do something that would let me have that feeling every day.

When I announced to my family that I was heading to culinary school in Paris after college, their reaction was not exactly ecstatic, but to their credit, they kept their doubts (mostly) to themselves. And a good thing, too, because there were plenty of days when I returned to my tiny Parisian apartment, exhausted from a day of babysitting soufflés and folding puff pastry, wondering exactly what I was doing there! But the pride I felt when I received my certification from Le Cordon Bleu gave me the confidence to know I had what it took to make it as a chef.

When I returned to Los Angeles and began working in restaurants, and then later as a private chef and caterer, I gained new insights into the way food impacts us every day. I saw how a good meal could turn a bad day around, and how a simple occasion could be elevated into a memorable one, all through food. I would happily have continued down that path indefinitely if Food Network hadn't come calling and offered me the chance to bring my distinctly Californian take on Italian cooking to a wider audience. Growing up in a family of filmmakers and actors, I'd never seen myself as a performer, much less a "personality," but when those opportunities present themselves, we owe it to ourselves to make the most of them. For twenty years, I had the privilege of coming into people's homes in a different way, sharing everything I'd learned about cooking—and learning what kind of dishes my audience loved best.

Three years ago, I pivoted again, this time into the world of food retail. With my website, Giadzy, I've been able to continue and expand upon the legacy of my grandfather Dino, getting back to the fundamentals and introducing quality Italian ingredients to this country in a different way, with a much greater reach than my grandfather was able to have with his two stores back in the day before e-commerce. Spreading the word about Italian culture

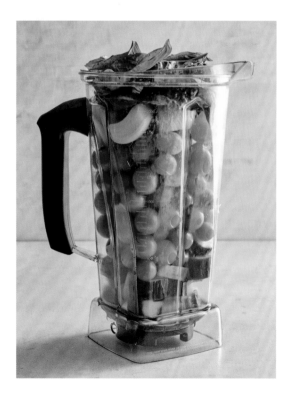

I am EXCITED to be focusing more than ever before on the power of INGREDIENTS.

and artisanal products is so important to me. Immersing myself in these unique foods has brought me closer to where I'm from and who I am, connecting the dots between me and my family. And I feel more myself than I ever have before.

Through it all, everything I've done in the food space has reflected one fundamental formula: Good Cooking = Technique + Ingredients + Ambience. And as a woman now in my fifties, I find that health needs to be part of that equation as well. If my years of cooking on TV primarily represented the technique part of the equation, and my catering and restaurant years were all about creating an ambience through food, I am excited to be focusing more than ever before on the power of ingredients. It's my goal with this book to show how choosing your ingredients wisely and well is the starting point not just to better meals, but to better health.

AFTER TEN BOOKS, SITTING down to start a cookbook is a bit daunting. Do I really have anything new to say? Haven't people gotten more recipes from me than they could possibly cook in a lifetime? But when I started to gather recipes for this book I realized that there have been some shifts in the way I cook today, a subtly different approach that has made me a smarter and, more important, a healthier cook. Every cookbook is a snapshot in time, and the pandemic changed the way we think about cooking and how we relate to food. These pivots, some small, some larger, are what this book is all about.

When I wrote my first health-focused cookbook, *Eat Better, Feel Better,* I was, frankly, not in a great place healthwise. I was working and traveling nonstop and any free time I managed to steal from my work obligations was devoted to my then-preteen daughter, Jade. Eventually the stress, quickly snatched meals, endless cups of coffee and sugary sweets for energy, and lack of anything resembling self-care took their toll on my digestion, my overall wellness—even my mental health. I was plagued by inflammation, I was always sick, and my digestion? It was just a straight-up mess. My approach to food needed a total reset and some fairly rigid guidelines to help me right the ship. And the philosophy I documented in *Eat Better, Feel Better* did the trick.

Today, I have enhanced my immunity, enhanced my health, and re-embraced my culture and heritage, all through food. These changes have unquestionably improved my quality of life overall. I'm happy to say I rarely have the kind of digestive woes and endless rounds of illness and infections I battled before I put my own health needs on the front burner. I still do a cleanse every so often, especially after the holidays or an indulgent vacation, and when I feel a need to course-correct, I return to the nutritional guidelines that helped me take control of my diet and digestive health. Once I'm back on track, I am able to spend more time thinking about what I should (and want to) eat, and less about what I shouldn't. On a day-to-day basis, I'm now a lot more relaxed about counting carbs or avoiding sugar than I needed to be when I was on a more restrictive regimen. I want to enjoy every bite and I want you to do the same. I just make sure that every bite I take carries the kind of wholesome, nutritionally dense ingredients that make me feel great. Most of all, I want to make every meal a joyful eating

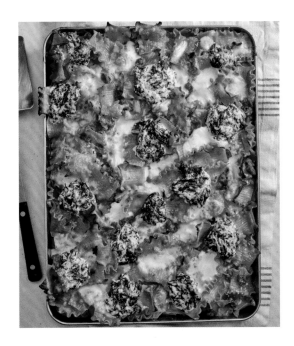

experience, because if the last few years have taught us anything, we can't take these moments for granted. That's the core of La Dolce Vita, and it's the Super-Italian way.

When Covid shut down my world for five or six months, it gave me the space to take a close look at my life and refocus my priorities. Today I am doing the things I've always wanted to do: opening more restaurants, forging new partnerships, and of course expanding my website, Giadzy. My attitudes about how much work to take on, and how much to travel, have really changed. Now that I no longer have a small child at home, I go back to Italy several times a year, and I got off the treadmill of filming television series several times a year. As a person in my fifties, I am excited about this time of life. I don't fear aging, but I want to make sure I can spend the years ahead as an active, inquisitive, robust old broad, ready to take on the next challenge, and navigate any pivots life throws at me with grace. Living and cooking the Super-Italian way is helping me do just that, and I hope it will do the same for you.

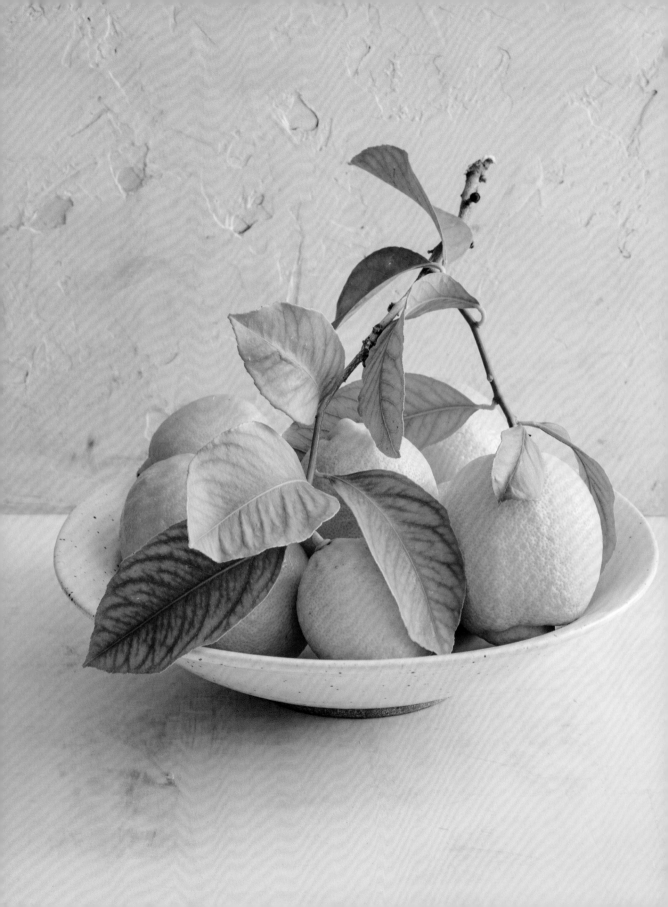

HARNESSING
the Goodness of
Authentic Italian Foods

LET'S FACE IT: We all know which foods don't actively contribute to good health. You don't need me to tell you that eating a lot of refined sugar and saturated fats and drinking alcohol to excess are not going to help you meet your wellness goals, whatever they may be.

And yet, living out our lives denying ourselves the opportunity to toast a friend's wedding, have a cupcake on a child's birthday, or enjoy the inimitable crunchy pleasure of biting into a fried calamari ring is not the perfect prescription for a life well lived. (As someone once said, eating a diet dictated solely by health concerns doesn't actually make you live longer, it just feels that way!)

Sad to say we probably all know a lot more about the "bad" things found in a lot of the foods we eat than the good stuff. Carbs, saturated fats, gluten, preservatives, and chemical additives, not to mention sugar in all its many forms, have all been excoriated by the media, nutritional "experts," even the health industry in recent years. There's a reason for that: Many of the diseases that plague us as we age can be traced to diets too full of these harmful ingredients, along with genetics and lifestyle.

But if food can cause inflammation, weight gain, and other maladies that lead to chronic illness, the flip side is equally true. A diet rich in micronutrients—the vitamins and minerals your body needs to stay strong and function properly—as well as antioxidants that tame inflammation, protein to help your body repair cells and make new ones, and fiber to keep your gut happy and remove waste, can make a world of difference in how you look and feel. You can add these key nutrients to your diet in the form of supplements (and I absolutely augment my diet to ensure I get enough of everything I need), but science is fairly united on the fact that getting as many nutrients as you can from the food you eat is the body's first and best line of defense.

For one thing, the nutrients found in food are often more potent than the kind you can pop in a capsule, whether plant- or animal-derived or synthetic (that is, manufactured in a lab). For another, nature is way ahead of the vitamin industrial complex when it comes to making the nutrients in your food readily available for use by your body during the digestive process, and to ensuring that you get a variety of nutrients at once, unlike single-nutrient pills. It's also much harder to overconsume a particular nutrient when it comes through food. Of course, the most obvious benefit to getting your nutrients from the end of a fork rather than out of a bottle is *taste*. Turns out that the things that are good for you are also the most delicious. Nature is smart that way.

And so are Italian cooks, who have a long tradition of eating in a more nutrient-dense way than most Americans. When Southern Italian cooks incorporate anchovies or colatura (a potent condiment made from anchovies) into dishes, it's a healthier, less fatty way to add flavor than loading them down with cheese or salt. Finishing off a soup with a drizzle of oil or fortifying a pasta dish with olives or a nutty pesto contributes a little good fat to an already healthful dish, *and* it benefits your hair, skin, and nails. Italians have been cooking this way for centuries, and it's something that my parents always reinforced throughout my childhood.

Now I am making a concerted effort to adopt this approach in my kitchen, and that's where my superfoods come in. This term has certainly gotten a workout in the past decade and often signifies foods with a near mythical ability to simultaneously lower your cholesterol and nourish your gut flora, tame inflammation, and boost immunity. The label has been slapped on everything from blueberries and salmon to kale and quinoa, as well as some fringier foods like adaptogens, açaí, and lion's mane mushrooms. While there is truth to many of these claims, the other, less often invoked truth is that the quantities of these foods you would need to consume is many times what most of us are likely to eat on any given day. (When was the last time you ate a cup of goji berries or chia seeds?) They are still excellent, healthful foods that deserve a place in your diet, they are just not exactly the miracle workers they are touted to be.

The items on my list of superfoods are similarly healthful and nutrient-dense, with more than their fair share of good fats, phytonutrients, and gut-pleasing fiber. That already puts them firmly in the dietary plus column. But for me, what truly vaults them into the superfood category is their ability to make *other* foods—the foods that make up the bulk of our diets, like lean proteins, whole grains, a variety of fruits and vegetables—downright craveable *and* give them a nice little nutritional boost while they're at it.

The foods listed starting on page 17 illustrate this quality perfectly. Without exception, these foods contribute needed nutrients and irresistible flavor to meals that you will look forward to eating every single day. But tasting good isn't enough; if it were, we could all look like a million bucks on a steady diet of chips and chocolate. To make my list of Super-Italian ingredients, a food needs to have hidden superpowers that help us stay strong, healthy, and well.

Turns out the things that are GOOD FOR YOU are also the most DELICIOUS.

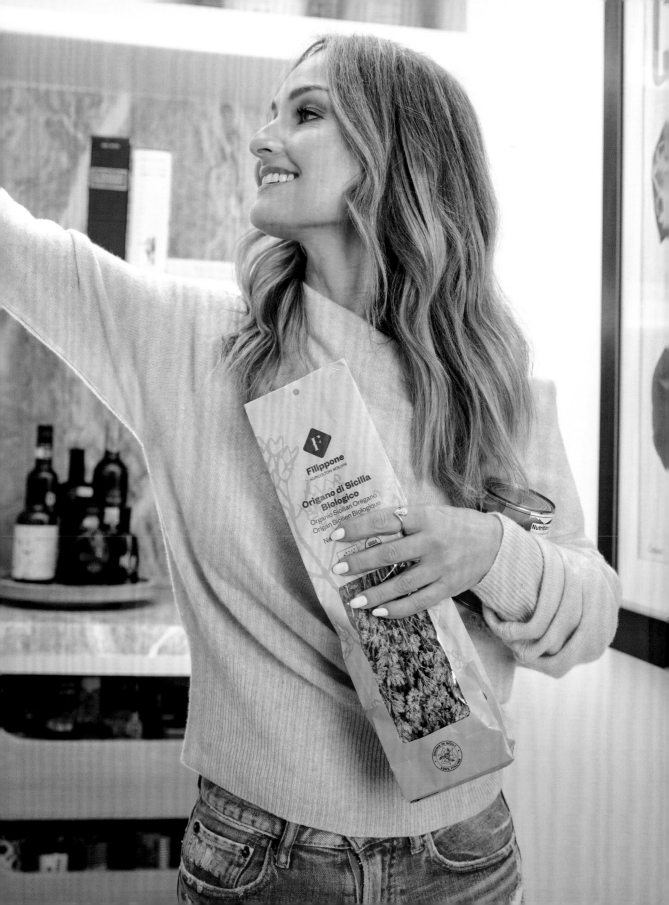

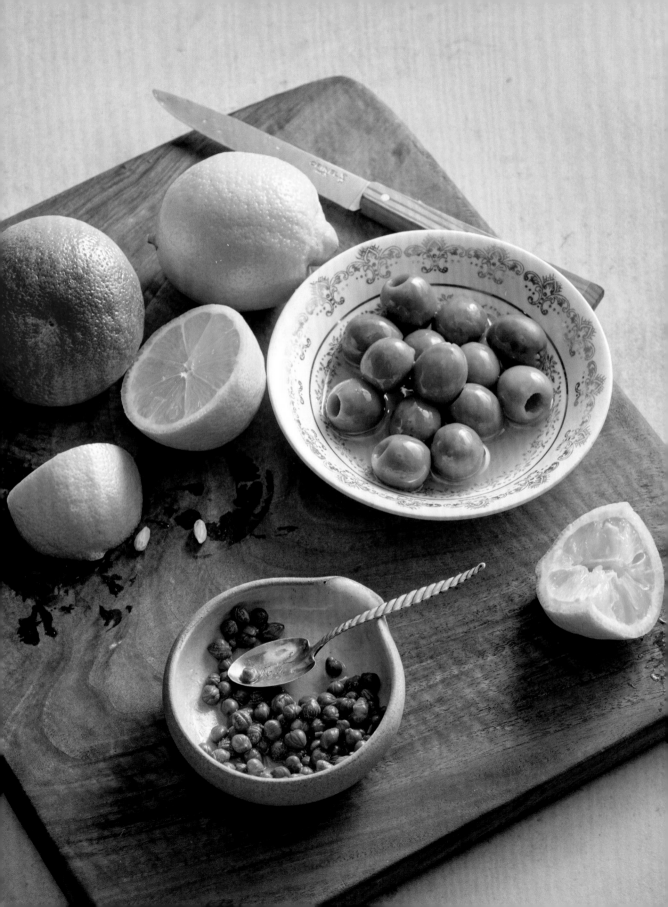

My Superfoods

The foods on the list that follows are my secret weapons for boosting the nutrition of everything I cook, and you will see them popping up often in the recipes. As I noted earlier, the ingredients that make my list are not only good for you, they also make things *taste* better, so that eating the things you *know* you should eat—lean proteins, seasonal fruits and vegetables, unprocessed and unrefined grains—is that much more pleasurable. These are the ingredients that I rely on to make every meal I serve nutritionally dense, supportive of my health, and incredibly delicious. I can't remember the time I made a recipe that didn't include at least three or four (and that's not even counting olive oil!), and the more I eat them, the more I love them. Better still, they love me back! So, without further ado, meet the superheroes of my Super-Italian kitchen:

1. Olives and Olive Oil

If I had to choose a desert island ingredient, it would hands down be olive oil (well, maybe chocolate and olive oil if I could have two). I use it for everything from cooking to skin care and I have been starting my day with a bowl of oatmeal topped with a few tablespoons of gorgeous extra-virgin olive oil for decades.

SUPERPOWERS ◆ Olives and the oils derived from them are full of "good fats," especially oleic acid, and a good source of antioxidants like vitamin E. Though depending on how the olives are preserved, they may be high in sodium.

FIND THEM IN ◆ Basically every recipe in this book, including Kale Salsa Verde (page 54), Umbrian Chicken Stew with Green Olives (page 163), and Grilled Swordfish with Olive Bagna Cauda (page 189).

2. Beans and Legumes

Beans are not a fixture in American homes the way they are throughout much of the rest of the world. Here we might throw them into a soup or chili, but they are rarely the star of the show. Italians, on the other hand, love beans, especially in the North, where they are served on their own as a side dish, often very simply prepared, the way we might serve roasted or mashed potatoes. Cannellini and lentils are probably the best known of the Italian beans, but cranberry, fava, and butter beans are all popular and delicious. I didn't eat a ton of beans growing up, but now I consider them a great addition to dishes when I want to add creaminess without dairy, or protein without meat. Whenever possible, I cook them from dried, but if time doesn't allow, canned is a good alternative, or frozen in the case of favas.

SUPERPOWERS ◆ Beans and legumes are a great source of fiber and a cheap, easy way to boost protein in all kinds of dishes, from soups to salads to pastas. The "tooty" effect of beans, the result of insoluble fiber fermenting in your digestive system (sorry!), is something your gut will adjust to over time, so build up slowly and beans won't give you any problems.

FIND THEM IN ◆ Artichoke Dip with White Beans (page 82), Siena-Style Ribollita (page 95), and Creamy Cannellini Beans (page 239), among others.

3. Cruciferous Vegetables

Dark, leafy, bitter greens are a major part of my diet. I like them, my body likes them—I just need them. Cruciferous veggies like escarole, dandelion greens, and broccoli rabe have always been the workhorses of Italian cuisine, the things that filled our plates and stomachs, supplemented by a small amount of meat. As a cook, I appreciate the way they have real presence on the plate and maintain their integrity without becoming too soft. These days I'm especially partial to Swiss chard (the rainbow variety is so pretty!), but broccoli rabe, Brussels sprouts, Tuscan kale, and cauliflower are all constant fixtures on my table—I never create a menu, even just for Jade and me, that doesn't include at least one kind of green, preferably two or more! I even use arugula the way other people use rice or noodles, as a bed for meat and fish as well as salads. As many of us gravitate toward a more vegetable-forward way of eating, these healthy plants have become increasingly popular, so it behooves us to learn how to cook them properly, and if I have anything to say about it, cruciferous vegetables in all their beautiful variety are going to be your new best friends.

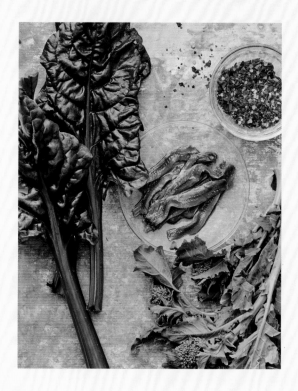

SUPERPOWERS ◆ Calorie for calorie, you can't get much more nutritional bang per bite than you will from a dark leafy green. Though their nutritional contents vary from variety to variety, they are all amazing sources of fiber; antioxidants; minerals, including iron, potassium, and magnesium; and vitamins like A, C, and K. Their high fiber content helps slow digestion and regulate blood sugar. And I just can't get enough of their vibrant, slightly bitter flavor.

FIND THEM IN ◆ Soooo many of these recipes! Check out Winter Beans and Greens Soup (page 91), Kale Salsa Verde (page 54), Orecchiette with Almond Pesto and Broccoli Rabe (page 128), and Siena-Style Ribollita (page 95).

4. Small Fish

Italians, especially those who live in the South, love their seafood and eat it far more often than Americans, who tend to draw the line at salmon and shrimp. No disrespect to those two (and you'll find plenty of ways to cook both in this book), but the very thing that makes them so popular in the

United States is what they lack: oils. Italians, by contrast, really prize small, oily fish like sardines, anchovies, and mackerel, and these small fish also happen to be more nutritionally dense than their leaner, bigger brethren. For one thing, the oils (essential fatty acids like omega-3 and omega-6) are great for us, and because the smaller fish spend very little time in the ocean, they have less exposure to the downside of the ocean in terms of heavy metals. They are also far more sustainable than bigger fish and less prone to icky things like parasites. Anchovies were a fixture in our kitchen when I was a kid, and lately I've gone a little anchovy crazy, adding them to dressings, stews, and pastas as an underlying layer of flavor.

SUPERPOWERS ◆ Small as they are, anchovies and other small fish are full of protein, essential fatty acids, and vitamins A and D. The bones in little fish, which become soft enough to eat during the canning process, are a good source of calcium.

FIND THEM IN ◆ Anchovies add their briny flavor to Garlicky Bread Crumbs (page 47), Caesar Aioli (page 53), and many, many more (shhhh, I won't tell if you don't). Try Pasta Assassina (page 141) for a good way to sample sardines.

5. Mushrooms

Mushrooms add a woodsy, meaty component to many Italian dishes, particularly in the North, where they are a staple ingredient. They are a great replacement for meat because they love aggressive seasoning, so they can be really flavorful, and I love the texture they add. We used dried porcini a lot when I was a kid because we couldn't get fresh ones in this country, and my mother would often pulverize them and use them as a base for stocks, sauces, and stews, a tip I use myself to enrich soups and simmered dishes. Many markets now offer a wide variety of fresh mushrooms—including exotic-looking maitake, trumpet, lion's mane, oyster, and shiitake—in addition to button mushrooms and creminis, all of which have different textures and flavors. Get a blend if you can and experiment with different types.

SUPERPOWERS ◆ Thanks in part to farmers' markets, where mushroom growers have been instrumental in introducing shoppers to a wider variety of mushrooms and educating them on the health benefits of their wares, mushrooms have become nutritional darlings in the past decade. And with good reason: This low-fat, high-fiber food has a fair amount of protein and minerals and is considered antioxidant, antiviral, anti-inflammatory, and cancer-fighting. Mushrooms' high concentration of probiotic insoluble fiber makes them useful in treating "bad" bacterial growth in the gut.

FIND THEM IN ◆ Beef and Porcini Stracotto (page 173), Rosemary Lentil Soup with Porcini (page 90), Mushroom-Stuffed Mushrooms (page 77), and Polenta with Braised Mushrooms (page 211).

6. Garlic

The pungent waft of garlicky aroma has come to be associated with Italian food, especially Italian American dishes created by immigrants in the early 1900s, but in Italy, garlic is both milder and used with much more restraint. Unless it is the main component of a dish, like garlic soup, Italians use garlic more as a flavor enhancer than as a flavor in its own right. I have a love-hate relationship with garlic. I don't digest it very well, but I love the taste. I also think garlic can very easily dominate and a little goes a long way. I prefer to season with garlic by smashing the whole peeled cloves to release their oils and using them to infuse their flavor into a dish, then discarding the cloves rather than eating a big bite of garlic.

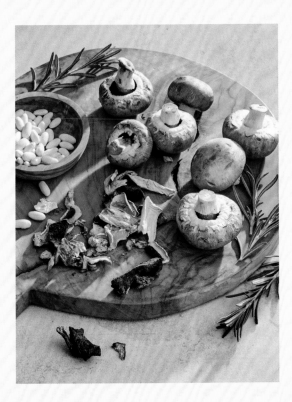

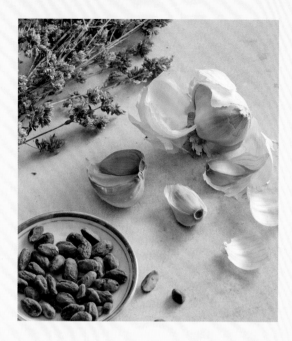

and appealing crunch they bring to my recipes. Nuts are strongly flavored, so you get a lot of bang for your buck. (Speaking of which, you might notice I haven't used pignolis in this book, both because their price has soared and because they have more fat than other nuts.)

SUPERPOWERS ◆ The fact that so many people have gravitated to nut-based milks and cheeses is proof of our growing appreciation for the health benefits of nuts. They are thought to help fight aging and have antioxidant properties, as well as providing protein and fiber.

FIND THEM IN ◆ Sicilian Pesto (page 60), Warm Farro with Mushrooms and Brussels Sprouts (page 240), and Apulian Almond Cookies (page 246).

8. Capers

Nothing else tastes quite like a caper, which is at once vegetal, briny, and earthy. The small capers we use most often (sometimes labeled nonpareil) are actually immature flower buds from the caper bush, but the larger, milder berries and even the leaves of the bush are also harvested and preserved to use as flavorings and garnishes. Like anchovies, capers add salinity to a dish but with more dimension than you get from pure salt. Some of the best are grown on a remote island called Pantelleria as well as in and around Sicily. Traditionally they were preserved in salt, which results in chewier capers with more concentrated flavor. Salt-cured capers need to be rinsed before using or they will be too overpowering, but the flavor is very pure. Less intense are brine-cured capers. The brine breaks down the capers a bit so they are softer and the flavor is milder; you can use the brine to flavor sauces and dressings.

SUPERPOWERS ◆ One of the oldest known plants used as medicine, garlic contains more than two hundred phytochemicals that endow it with all the "anti" properties: anti-cancer, anti-inflammatory, antifungal, antimicrobial, antidiabetic, and more. Some people, including me, find it hard to digest, but if you love garlic and do really well with it, eat up. It has healing properties and aids digestion.

FIND IT IN ◆ Pretty much everywhere but the dessert chapter!

7. Nuts

I have long been a fan of nuts as a healthy, easily portable snack, and I rarely leave the house without a stash of almonds in my bag. But while almonds are used in Italian cooking, other varieties are far more popular there. Hazelnut trees are often grown near olive groves, as they are complementary growing partners, and Sicily is world renowned for its bright green, flavorful pistachios. Both show up often in Italian dishes and I've been loving the more distinctive flavors

SUPERPOWERS ◆ These tiny dynamos are considered a good source of antioxidants, as well as nutrients like vitamin K, B vitamins, minerals like iron and calcium, and chemicals that help regulate blood sugar. Keep in mind, however, that they are a high-sodium food.

FIND THEM IN ◆ Kale Salsa Verde (page 54), Chicken Piccata Meatballs (page 160), and Crunchy Baked Sole with Capers (page 196).

9. Chiles

Chiles elevate sensation like nothing else, opening our taste buds (and sinuses!) and causing a physical reaction. Traditionally heat was used to mask less pleasant flavors and to cool off the body in warm climates; today we use chiles to add a dimension of flavor to things that are flat or bland. Calabrian chile paste, which is made of chopped chiles that have been sun-dried and marinated in oil, is my go-to for infusing a little fire into dishes because it adds a bit of sweetness as well as heat, but I use red pepper flakes, too. I like chiles best when they remain in the background; a straight kick in the mouth with heat is not the way I like to taste food, but to each their own!

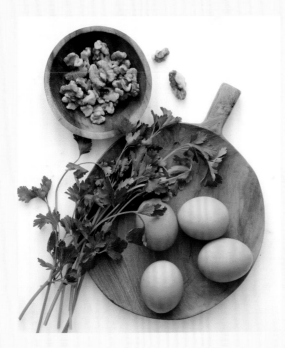

SUPERPOWERS ◆ Many of the benefits of chiles can be traced to their high concentration of capsaicin, the compound that gives them their heat and also has been proved to fight heart disease and cancer and to boost metabolism. Their generous concentration of antioxidants like vitamin C makes them immunity boosters.

FIND THEM IN ◆ Calabrian Chile Garlic Oil (page 50), Pork Scarpariello (page 168), and Calabrian Pomodoro (page 61).

10. Vinegar

From a culinary perspective, all dishes need an element of acid; it's essential to balancing flavors, and without it food can taste flat and one-dimensional. Like a squeeze of citrus, a dash of vinegar brings out flavor; next time you think your food needs salt, try adding a hit of acid first. You'll see how it wakes up heavy, hearty dishes like meat stews and salads of sturdy greens. Italians use a range of vinegars in their cooking, from the relatively mild tang of balsamic and white wine vinegars to the stronger, more rustic red wine vinegars. I also keep apple cider vinegar on hand when I want a sweet-sour taste.

SUPERPOWERS ◆ In addition to being a preservative, vinegar has antifungal and antibacterial properties. When I was pregnant with Jade, someone told me if I had heartburn, a teaspoon of vinegar would settle my stomach, though I never tested the theory.

FIND IT IN ◆ Balsamic Chocolate Truffles (page 251).

11. Citrus

My love of citrus is well documented, and in my opinion, there are few dishes that don't benefit from a squeeze of lemon juice or a quick grating of zest. Like a dash of vinegar, citrus wakes up flavors, but it's less pungent, so it won't overwhelm delicate foods like fish and tender greens. I love the fact that you can use the whole fruit: juice, rind, and all. You'll find amazing citrus fruit growing throughout Southern Italy, not only lemons, but oranges, tangerines, and citrons, so my appreciation of all things citrus definitely comes naturally!

SUPERPOWERS ◆ All citrus fruits are low-calorie foods rich in vitamins (notably vitamin C) and antioxidants. Their vitamin C content aids in the absorption of other nutrients from foods, like iron, and has been connected to the prevention of cancer and kidney stones and to boosting immunity.

FIND IT IN ◆ GDL Seasoned Salt (page 48), Lemon Affogato (page 265), and Grilled Endive Salad with Citrus and Pancetta (page 103).

12. Herbs

The aroma of a dish is a huge part of its appeal, and nothing adds more enticing aroma than herbs, whether fresh or dried. Basil is probably the herb most associated with Italian cooking, but oregano, mint, parsley, and rosemary are all used to add flavor, color, and fragrance to dishes from north to south. Living in California, I am able to keep an herb garden growing year-round, but I augment the fresh herbs with dried herbs imported from Italy, in particular Sicilian oregano. It has a unique flavor that is a direct expression of Sicily's terroir, a combination of rich volcanic soil and sea air. There oregano is dried and packaged on the stems. It's deliciously herby with a hint of sweetness, and so perfumed you don't need a lot of it.

SUPERPOWERS ◆ Benefits vary from one variety to another, but all herbs are low in calories, high in fiber, and universal flavor enhancers. Some, like parsley, have a nice amount of vitamins A, C, and K as well as iron, and basil is full of antioxidants; both can be added to salads as a green. Mint and oregano are thought to have antimicrobial properties.

FIND THEM IN ◆ GDL Seasoned Salt (page 48), Parmesan Basil Butter (page 56), and Basil Panna Cotta with Strawberries (page 261).

13. Eggs

Now that we understand that eggs don't really contribute to high cholesterol or heart disease (saturated fats are far greater culprits), they are back on the menu in a big way and with good reason. They just might be the ultimate convenience food, there at the ready for a quick and easy pantry meal any time of day. They are an excellent source of protein for anyone looking to reduce the amount of meat in their diet. Even before she became largely vegetarian, my mother made eggs for dinner often, using them to transform leftovers into a frittata, spaghetti "pizza," or stuffed crepes. As with meat, knowing where and how your eggs were produced matters; whenever possible, choose eggs from humanely raised chickens fed an organic diet.

SUPERPOWERS ◆ Beyond protein, eggs provide vitamins D, A, and B_{12}. They are also a good source of folate, important for pregnant women and their babies.

FIND THEM IN ◆ Green Stracciatella (page 88), Baked Egg Crepe Casserole (page 218), Skillet Eggs with Bread Crumbs (page 215), and Caesar Aioli (page 53).

14. Tomatoes

Fresh, dried, canned, or pureed, tomatoes are the backbone of so many foods we equate with Italian cooking—pretty amazing considering they are not even native to Europe and didn't find their way into Italian kitchens until four or five hundred years ago. (That may sound like a long time, but remember there are ruins in Rome dating back to the eighth century BC!) At once sharp and sweet, tomatoes add brightness, depth, and that savory flavor known as umami to just about every kind of dish, from sauces to salads.

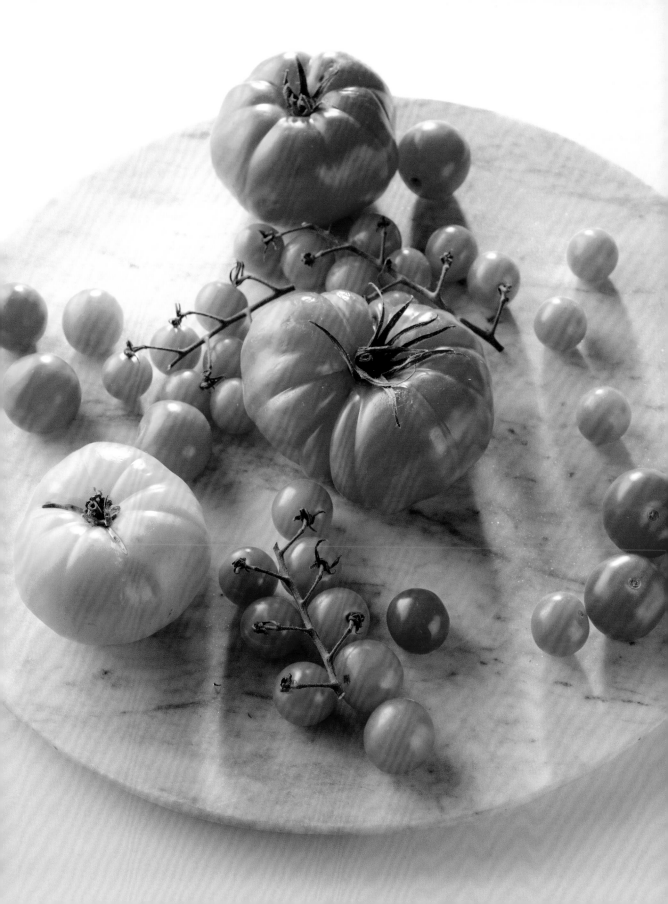

SUPERPOWERS ◆ Tomatoes of all kinds are low in calories, have a decent amount of fiber, and are a good source of vitamins A and C. They are a particularly good source of lutein, an antioxidant thought to help prevent cancer, as well as lycopene and beta-carotene.

FIND THEM IN ◆ Plenty of the pastas in Chapter 4 (page 111) as well as Umbrian Chicken Stew with Green Olives (page 163), Tomatoes Gratinata (page 235), and Sicilian Pesto (page 60).

15. La Dolce Vita

This is the one item on this list that you can't buy from a store. A joyful approach to cooking and eating is as essential to good food as salt and pepper, and very much a part of Italian culture. It may sound trite, but when you cook with love and have fun in the kitchen, the food just *tastes* better. Anxiety should not govern the way any of us interacts with food; we need to live our lives and have fun doing it. Be honest about who you are and what you like. Eat everything, but do it mindfully. And when you cook, try not to put too much pressure on yourself. Bring other people into the kitchen, and if someone offers to contribute to a meal, let them. If it's not perfect, so what? No one expects a five-star meal—that's why we go to restaurants! Just cook something you like and look forward to eating, and everyone else will, too. Above all, remember that every meal is an opportunity for pleasure. People enjoy spending time with someone who is relaxed and happy more than they do with someone exhausted or exasperated. Don't dwell on what didn't come out exactly the way you hoped and focus on how much fun everyone is having. Take time to enjoy these moments of shared pleasure around the table, because they are fleeting.

SUPERPOWERS ◆ A wonderful meal not only nourishes the body, it releases endorphins, nourishing the mind and soul.

FIND IT IN ◆ Every single one of the recipes in this book. Buon appetito!

To make sure you always have these superfoods easily at hand, I've created a whole arsenal of ready-to-use condiments and flavor enhancers, each of them packed with Super-Italian ingredients. I strongly recommend that you check out Chapter 1: Flavor Starts Here (page 43) and set aside a bit of time to make a few—or all—of them! They are the best way I know to make weeknight dinners or informal gatherings an absolute breeze without having to resort to prepared foods and other not-so-great-for-you shortcuts. Making liberal and frequent use of these condiments and the superfoods they contain is a big part of how I think about food now. Read on for more about how I have subtly modified my approach to cooking as I prioritize health, balance, and pleasure in the kitchen.

KEY NUTRIENTS

	Protein	Vitamins	Fiber	Good Fats	Antioxidants	Minerals	Superpowers
Olives/ olive oil	✓	✓ Especially vitamin E	✓ (In whole olives)	✓	✓		Oleic acid may reduce cholesterol
Beans	✓		✓		✓	✓ Especially iron, potassium, and magnesium	More protein than most plant-based foods
Cruciferous vegetables	✓	✓	✓		✓	✓	Vitamin K, good for blood and bone health
Small fish	✓	✓		✓		✓	The omega-3 fatty acids in fish may help prevent heart disease
Mushrooms	✓	✓	✓		✓	✓	Immune boosters and anti-inflammatory
Garlic					✓	✓	Antiviral, antibacterial, and antifungal properties—it may even prevent the common cold
Nuts	✓	✓	✓	✓	✓	✓	Have been associated with weight loss, despite relatively high calorie content
Capers	✓	✓	✓		✓	✓	The richest source of quercetin, a powerful antioxidant
Chiles		✓	✓		✓		Can reduce the effects of acid reflux
Vinegar					✓		Considered a disinfectant and can kill bacteria
Citrus		✓	✓ (When eaten as whole fruit)		✓	✓	Vitamin C strengthens the immune system
Herbs		✓	✓		✓		Plant-based polyphenols protect against a host of illnesses, including cancer
Eggs	✓	✓					Choline supports a healthy memory
Tomatoes		✓	✓				The lycopene in tomatoes may protect against sunburn.

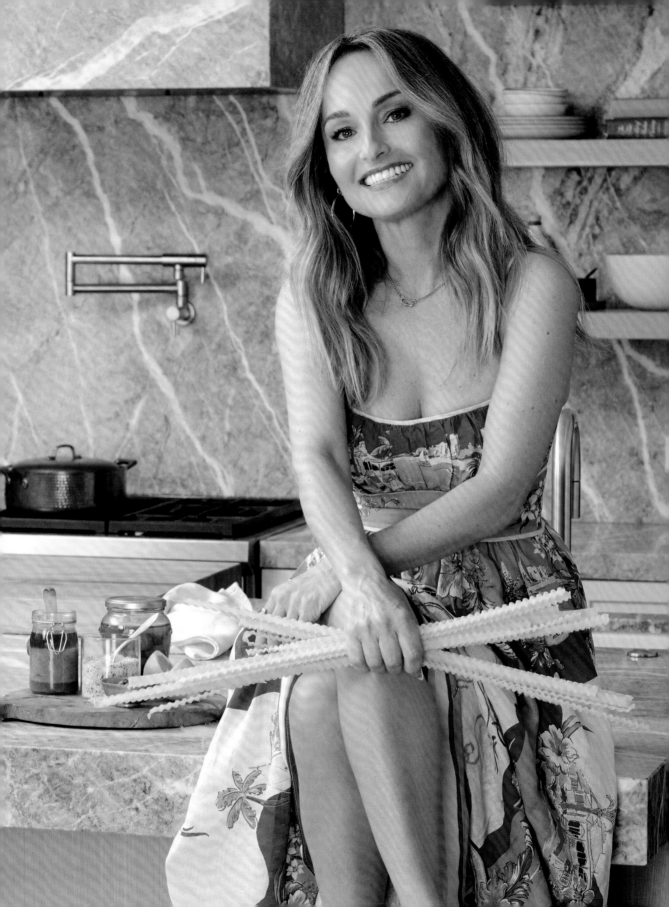

COOKING THE

Super-Italian Way:

How I Cook Now

IF I HAD to single out the biggest change to the way I cook today versus how I cooked a decade ago, it would be more emphasis on ingredients and a better understanding of how they make me feel when I eat them. I've come to realize that it's hard to make a bad dish if you start with truly delicious, excellent components, simply assembled and prepared, while even the most accomplished chef wizardry can't really create a masterpiece from so-so building blocks. Maybe it's a return to my roots, or maybe as a working parent I simply no longer have the patience to bother with tweezers and mandolines and the like, but I've found the more I pare down my recipes and let each element truly shine, the happier I am in the kitchen—and at the table.

This shift really started when I began traveling to Italy on a more regular basis, both to get back in touch with my roots after four decades in the United States and to enjoy the slower pace of life that Italians embrace. I noticed right away that some of the stomach issues that gave me trouble at home just didn't seem to bother me in Italy. The food I was eating was minimally processed and prepared more simply, and my body loved it. Bottom line: I felt better when I ate in Italy.

When I got back home to the United States, I tried to find a trusted source for unadulterated products like those available everywhere in Italy, foods that were produced and packaged in the old ways. When I couldn't find one, it became my mission to be that source for others. Just as my grandfather Dino had (I love how life comes full circle sometimes), I began seeking out ingredients that never made their way onto

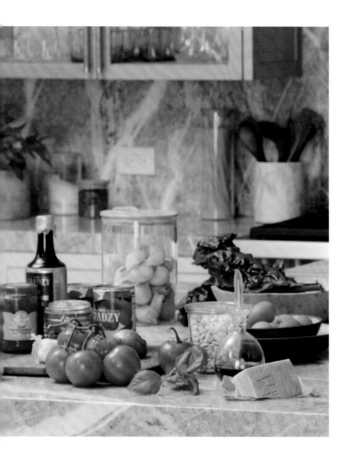

of where and how the olives are grown. It has been fascinating, and also an exciting new chapter in my life, getting to share these incredible ingredients with people.

This deep dive into ingredients has also taught me so much about health. When I started Giadzy, I thought that we could go with cheaper ingredients that are easier to access, but I soon came to realize these inferior products are just not as good for you. The rise in highly processed foods in our diet has led to a crisis in health, with illnesses once seen mostly in older people becoming more common among young people. The more processed our food is, the farther away we get from good health.

Whether you stock your pantry from my website, a local Italian market, or the grocery store down the street, I want to challenge you to make quality the first criterion when you put something in your cart, even if it means you buy less. When it comes to flavor, but perhaps even more crucially, when it comes to your health, quality is *everything*. Do a cleanse on your pantry: Look at the labels of what's on the shelf. Your pasta should contain semolina flour and not much else. How much sugar is in your pasta sauce? When shopping, read the labels, and if the ingredient list is longer than five or six items, keep moving. Know where your food comes from and what goes into it. Buy the best you can afford, and choose organic whenever possible. If you buy a lesser version you could end up eating more artificial coloring, additives, preservatives, sugar, and flavor enhancers. All these factors matter when you are cooking for good health and will bear dividends in the long run.

American shelves: things like fragrant Sicilian oregano, jarred sweet cherry tomatoes, dried caper leaves, unusual beans, and fun pasta shapes made with traditional bronze dies and real semolina flour. I traveled back to Italy frequently and while there spent time with artisanal producers from north to south. These small family operations were always eager to explain to me how the structure of the soil, the quality of the air and water, the local terroir all affect the quality of their products. I learned that Sicilian tomatoes that grow at the base of Mount Etna, without irrigation, taste completely different from San Marzano tomatoes, which come from the area outside Naples. I also learned that there is no such thing as "regular" olive oil; each one has a unique flavor that is an expression

Essentials of the Italian Pantry

For an Italian cook, the process of making a meal is just as important as the final outcome, and that process starts with shopping. In Italy, where few homes have the oversized fridges we do, and the tradition of visiting the butcher, fishmonger, and produce market is strong, it is common to shop every day and maintain a fairly minimal pantry. Cooks walk into food shops with an open mind, letting the season and what looks good in the market dictate what's for dinner.

Much as I would love to follow that relaxed approach to menu planning, I rarely have the bandwidth to shop that often. I do stock up on meat and fresh vegetables once or twice a week, but many of the meals I cook start with a trip to my pantry. Knowing I can get in and out of the market with just a few items on my list takes a lot of the stress out of mealtime. Even on the days when I don't have a second to shop, I've always got the makings of something healthy, wholesome, and fast within reach.

Side note: Unlike many people, I don't think of my freezer as an extension of my pantry. You won't find a lot in my freezer besides gelato, ice cream, a bag of frozen peas, and some potato puffs for Jade. If I make a big batch of tomato sauce, chicken broth, or cookie dough, I might set some aside for a later date; I also store my chocolate in the freezer to keep it fresh (and out of sight!). Otherwise, I like to cook and eat fresh food. But that's just me. The point is to cook with whole, unprocessed foods as much as possible, and in a way that works for you.

Many of the items on the list that follows also appear on my superfood rundown on page 25. That's not a coincidence; those nutrient-dense ingredients, as well as the condiments I love to make from them, are the cornerstones of nearly everything I cook these days. What follows are my tips for choosing the best of the best so that you can cook more flavorfully and simply every day. And visit my website, www.giadzy.com, for a deeper look at some of the exceptional artisanal

growers and small producers I've had the pleasure of meeting and learning from in my quest to discover the very best of Italian ingredients.

Olive oil

Olives are cultivated all throughout Italy, as well as in the greater Mediterranean region and beyond. The finest olive oils are monocultural, meaning they are made exclusively from olives grown in a specific region with a distinctive flavor reflecting that region. Most mass-marketed oils, in contrast, are a blend of oils from different regions and even different countries, combined to make a consistent, more neutral product. I've really come to appreciate the nuances that differentiate these oils. For instance, olives from the North of Italy and the oils pressed from them are quite mild, verging on buttery, while Southern olives are exposed to intense sun, Mediterranean salt air, and volcanic soil, all of which give them bolder flavors with a grassy or spicy aftertaste that lingers on your tongue. The only way to figure out which olive oil you prefer is to try a few. Make sure any you buy are extra-virgin and don't contain any seed oils or other extenders. Italians usually have several varieties on their kitchen shelves the way an American cook might have sesame or walnut or avocado oil in the pantry. When it comes to whole olives, I find green olives have a milder, fruitier flavor and firmer texture that I prefer to the softer, chewier brown and black olives. For most of my recipes, I prefer olives packed in brine to the drier, more leathery oil-cured ones.

MY PICKS ◆ For cooking I would use an oil from Liguria, which tends to be a little milder. For drizzling and other finishing uses I reach for a stronger flavored oil from Puglia or Sicily. Brine-cured green Castelvetrano olives are the ones I use most.

Tomatoes

San Marzano tomatoes get all the good press, but in my day-to-day cooking I usually reach for *passata*—a simple puree of tomatoes—or cherry tomatoes in a can or jar. I find them so much sweeter and more delicate in flavor, and they don't need to cook as long. Corbarini from Campagna, datterini from Puglia, and pomodorini from all over the South are all cultivated in Campagnia, just as San Marzanos are, but have way lower acidity.

MY PICKS ◆ I am never without several cans of sweet cherry tomatoes, jarred yellow *datterini* (translates to "little fingers"), squeeze tubes of tomato paste, and 24-ounce jars of passata.

Pasta

For most of my life, my family has imported our pasta; now it's possible to find good imported pasta made with very simple ingredients just about everywhere, and if there is one category I'd urge you to splurge on a bit, it's this one. Stocking up on bargain pastas may seem like a good way to economize, but you get what you pay for. Now that I have my own line of pastas, I can geek out on the topic all day, but whether you buy mine or another brand, the rules are the same: They should have minimal ingredients—ideally only semolina and water—and be cut

with bronze dies, which gives them a rough texture that grabs and holds the sauce. Mass-produced pastas contain very little semolina and are extruded through plastic dies so they are smooth and slippery. Not only that, but for many people with gluten sensitivities, pastas imported from Italy, made from Italian grain, may be tolerated better than pastas made from domestic grain—that's how different agriculture in the two countries is.

MY PICKS ◆ The pasta shapes we sell on Giadzy are the ones I grew up eating and remind me of my childhood. Some that I like to have on hand are a couple of short cuts like curly nodi marini and ruffle-edge taccole, as well as at least one long pasta, like a spaghetti chitarra or a bucatini.

Grains

They will never displace pasta in the Italian pantry, but even I like to mix it up now and then. Rice (white or brown), whole grains like farro, and fregola (technically a pasta, similar to couscous, that can be used like a grain) are all a nice change of pace, and in many cases can be used interchangeably in salads or risottos.

MY PICKS ◆ A short-grain Italian rice (I prefer Carnaroli, but Arborio is great, too) for risottos, farro for cold grain salads and "farrottos," and quick-cooking polenta are all standbys.

Vinegar

Modena has the best balsamic vinegar. You can spend a lot on balsamics, but I don't really think that's necessary; unless you are a balsamic connoisseur, you don't need one that is super aged for most day-to-day use.

MY PICKS ◆ One fairly neutral option, like apple cider vinegar, a red wine vinegar, and a balsamic.

Other pantry items

Panko bread crumbs, boxed low-sodium chicken broth (preferably organic, free-range), dried porcini mushrooms, oil-packed anchovies, colatura, tuna and sardines, capers, dried herbs (especially Sicilian oregano), Calabrian chile paste, red pepper flakes, and salt. (A note about salt: I cook exclusively with kosher salt—plus Maldon sea salt flakes for sprinkling on finished dishes. The salinity of kosher salt can vary from brand to brand, with Morton's generally considered to be "saltier" than Diamond Crystal kosher salt. The recipes in this book were developed using Diamond Crystal kosher salt, so if you use another brand, you may want to adjust the amount you add. As always, season to taste.)

Dairy

Unless you are lactose intolerant, there is no reason to avoid cooking with dairy as long as you don't go overboard. I find stirring a small amount of butter into a sauce right at the end makes it so much more indulgent. And aged hard cheeses like Parmesan and pecorino add a salty, yummy umami depth to dishes I just can't do without. Adding them later in the cooking process is almost like using a finishing salt. They are also good keepers, so they are easy to have on hand. Other cheeses—like Gorgonzola, ricotta, provolone—I generally buy on an as-needed basis, and only in the quantities I need to avoid waste.

MY PICKS ◆ Unsalted butter, of course, plus a block of Parmigiano-Reggiano cheese and Pecorino Romano or Pecorino Sardo are musts, not only for grating but for the flavor their rinds add to simmered dishes. They are also handy to put on a cheese platter . . . and for me to snack on while I'm cooking! I usually have a tub of either ricotta or mascarpone, but I rarely have both at the same time because they spoil relatively quickly.

Other fridge items

A hunk of pancetta (it can also live in the freezer), eggs, Dijon mustard, capers, lemons, fresh herbs (parsley, basil, mint), and at least one kind of bitter green (usually arugula).

Alliums

Onions, shallots, leeks, and garlic are all ubiquitous in Italian cuisine, and it's almost not worth starting to cook if you don't have at least one of these! That said, they are largely interchangeable; as long as you have some member of the allium family on hand, you should be covered.

MY PICKS ◆ Maybe it's my French training, but the sweeter flavor and milder bite of shallots make them a nonnegotiable and, of course, a head or two of fresh, sweet garlic.

Nuts

I go through a lot of nuts because I snack on them, add them to salads and pestos, and use them in baking. If you don't use nuts frequently, store them in the freezer to prevent them from becoming rancid. Much as pignolis are a fixture in Italian cuisine, their cost has become so high and they go bad so quickly that I buy them only on an occasional basis these days.

MY PICKS ◆ Almonds are my go-to nuts for every day, plus other nuts, like hazelnuts, pistachios, or walnuts, for baking.

Miscellaneous

Rice flour for dredging and coatings, all-purpose and almond flour for baking, chocolate for the obvious reasons.

My Cooking Mantras

As my approach to food has evolved over the years, so has the way I think about cooking. As I continue to reconnect with my Italian roots, I find myself adopting the practical approach to making meals I see in home kitchens all over Italy, and the respect cooks have for using and serving the best ingredients available to them. It's the way my grandparents and mother cooked, and it's the kind of cooking philosophy I hope to pass along to Jade as she gets closer to striking out on her own.

No Fake Foods

When I started pulling together the recipes for this book, I knew early on that I wanted to use only real, whole foods, even if it meant I couldn't use some of them quite as lavishly as I might have in the past. I'd rather have a little of something good than a lotta something "lite." That means full-fat ricotta, whole milk, pasta made from semolina wheat, and good chocolate and real sugar in my desserts. (Obviously if you have a health condition like celiac disease, you should follow your doctor's recommendations on eating gluten.) When I call for Parmesan, I mean a good, aged Parmigiano-Reggiano cheese, the kind that comes with the rind and that you grate yourself. Sure, it's a bit pricey, but you're going to make it go a long way and love every bite. I can't say it enough: Quality matters.

Learn to Love Leftovers

One major difference in the way Italians think about cooking is that they don't try to reinvent the wheel every day; they use leftovers to kick-start new meals. I'm not talking about our concept of leftovers, which usually just means reheating a portion of the previous day's lasagna or soup. A pragmatic Italian cook will make things like beans, sauces, and condiments in big quantities and then just eat them until they are used up. Take Peperonata (page 59) for example: One night it will be a side dish, another night a condiment for baked fish in parchment (page 201) or part of an antipasto spread. The same goes for Creamy Cannellini Beans (page 239), which stand on their own as a great side dish but can also be used as a bed for grilled meats or tossed with pasta for an instant sauce. It's an approach I've really been embracing as a way to take one task off the day's to-do list. Throughout this book I've given you some pointers for repurposing your leftovers, so think about making double batches and getting a leg up on meals down the line.

Texture Is Everything

I'll admit it, I crave the crunch. When foods are too soft, too same-same in texture without a bit of contrast to add interest, it's a hard pass for me. I need that crackle of toasted crumbs on my baked scallops, crave the crispy bits of frizzled cheese around the edges of my Layerless Sheet Pan Lasagna (page 135), need a handful of nuts or chopped romaine in my salads to make them more fun to chew. That's how I see food, and that's what makes my mouth water. Crispy, crunchy, golden-crusted—all of these are synonyms for delicious in my book, and I think most people agree that foods with a mixture of textures are just more satisfying to eat. Which is why . . .

I'd rather have a LITTLE of something GOOD than a lotta something "LITE."

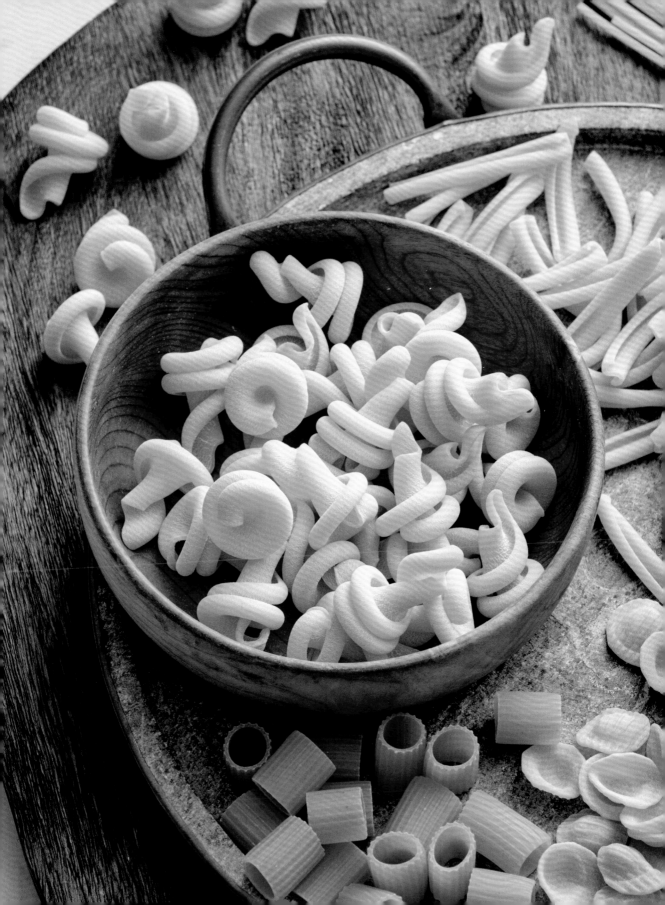

Heat Is Your Friend

Maybe it's because I have been spending more time at my restaurants, and restaurant chefs are notorious for letting it rip when it comes to cooking temperatures, but lately I have been harnessing the power of heat to help lock in flavor and create tempting textures in a lot of the meals I make. You'll see throughout this book that many recipes direct you to cook certain foods at high heat—not medium-high, but really high: 450°F or even higher in some instances! I find that a shorter cooking time at a higher temperature helps create a beautifully browned, crisp exterior on foods that seals in juices and just makes them look a lot more tempting.

Cooking at high heat also enables me to lean more heavily on my oven as a stand-in for frying. I find when I cook lightly oiled food on a preheated sheet pan at really high temps I get nice exterior browning and tender interiors without all the fat and greasiness that come with deep-frying. I use this technique for the eggplant in my version of pasta alla Norma, my chicken parm, and much more. The results aren't quite as crisp, but you still get plenty of satisfying crunch and it's a trade-off I'm happy to make for food that is lighter and more healthful. Another plus is that you won't end up with all that used oil to dispose of, making it a lot more economical!

High heat also helps me create a good, hard sear on foods when I'm pan-frying, as with Simple Seared Salmon on Minted Pea Puree (page 192). That crust not only adds plate appeal, it helps prevent the flesh from drying out. And I use my broiler to give a final blast of heat to brown the surfaces of many baked dishes and create that chewy cheesy crispy crust on things like my Layerless Sheet Pan Lasagna (page 135). So don't be timid when it comes to cranking up that dial all the way!

Let Condiments Do the Heavy Lifting

You know those nights when you stare blankly into the fridge, trying to get inspired to make something for dinner? (Yes, I promise you, I have plenty of those nights, too!) I can't tell you how many times it's been a condiment that jump-started the creative process for me. There is simply no easier way to elevate something pretty basic like a chicken breast or fish fillet into something that looks like you made a real effort—restaurant-worthy, even! A grilled chicken breast is a real snooze; grilled chicken with Kale Salsa Verde (page 54) or Green Olive Relish (page 55)? Now, that's something I would order off a menu any day. Yet if you have stocked up on the condiments and other basics on pages 43 to 65, the two chicken dishes will take **exactly the same amount of time to make!** If I can convince you to make one recipe in this book, it is the anchovy-scented Garlicky Bread Crumbs (page 47). These fragrant, crispy morsels instantly elevate any dish with a salty, savory little kick and make it look just a bit more finished. Add a sprinkle to a tried-and-true recipe and see if you don't agree they give it an instant upgrade.

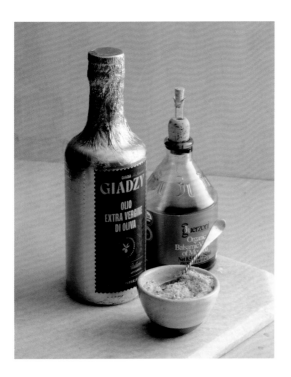

Use High-Carb and Calorie-Dense Foods Strategically

One of the real advantages of buying and cooking with top-quality ingredients is that you don't need to do a lot to them to make them taste amazing. I love the taste of Parmesan, and I use it (or pecorino) in many of the recipes in this book, but with a lot more restraint than I have in the past—almost as a seasoning, to add a nutty, salty note, rather than as the main flavor of a dish. Not only does it reduce the overall fat and calories, it allows the food it is paired with to shine more brightly.

Reduce Portion Size

It's not sexy, but it's a fact: Portion control is one of the primary ways I am able to indulge in all my favorite foods without ever truly dieting. In fact, I'd go so far as to say that moderation is the difference between dieting and dining. One is about avoidance and restriction, the other is about taking your pleasures in reasonable doses and enjoying every bite mindfully.

I won't pretend I'm one of those women with iron will who can take one bite of a dessert and push the rest away; I'm more likely to be scraping the bowl for every last bite! Plus, the idea of wasting food like that doesn't really sit well with me. I'd rather give myself (and everyone else, for that matter) a reasonable portion of pasta, meat, or dessert, and let them go back for seconds if they want. Nine times out of ten I find that people are satisfied with less than they have been conditioned to expect. That's why I suggest a pasta recipe made with 1 pound of pasta to easily serve 6 (or 4 with leftovers for tomorrow's lunch). And rather than making my desserts less luscious and indulgent, I just serve them up in smaller portions. I'm still scraping the bottom of the bowl. There's just a little less to scrape, but I feel like I got a full serving. It should go without saying, of course, that this rule does not apply to veggies or most salads, which you can and should eat as much of as you want; in those cases, my

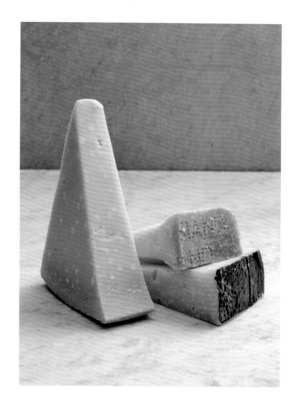

portions are far more generous, and may seem *too* big to you if you think of anything green as a plate filler. So . . .

Don't Skip the Salad

I consider salad an integral part of any meal, and I eat at least one, and often two, every single day. Not only do I like having something fresh and uncooked with my meal for the textural variety, but making sure that there are plenty of greens—especially of the dark leafy variety—is an ironclad guarantee that I will get plenty of the nutrients and fiber I need in my diet.

I hope these tips help you streamline your cooking routine and get the most out of every minute you spend in the kitchen—and at the table. I know cooking has come to feel so much more intuitive and rewarding to me since I adopted this approach, and I bet it will do the same for you!

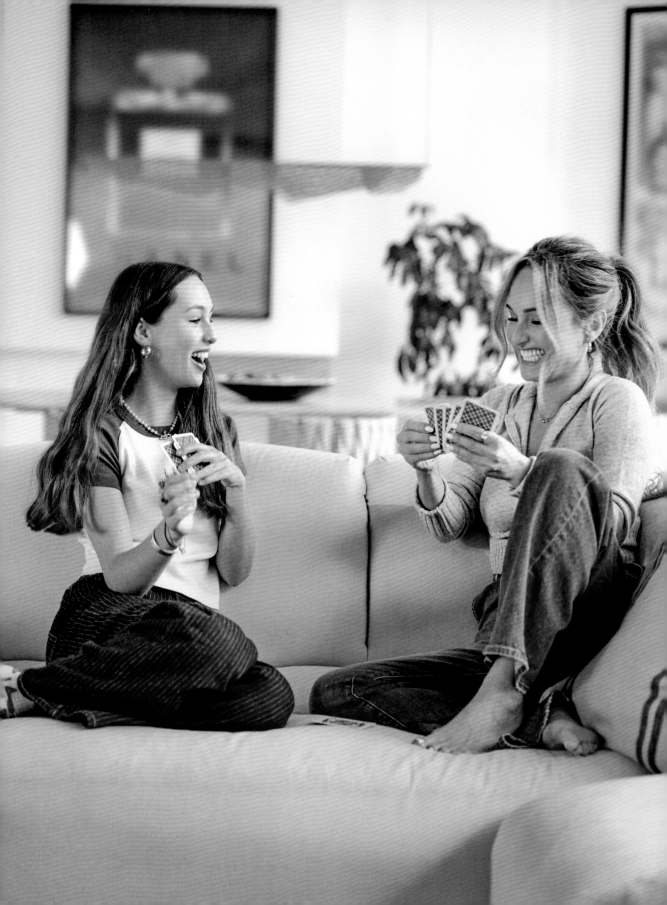

LIVING

La Dolce Vita:

A Balanced Approach to Wellness

WHAT WE EAT has a huge impact on how we feel, how we age, and, let's face it, how we look. But good health isn't only a reflection of the food we put in our bodies; genetics, environmental factors, and lifestyle choices all play their roles, too. Some of these are more within our control than others, but all make up a part of the puzzle that is wellness.

Let's tackle lifestyle first: You can eat like a Buddhist monk and still feel less than amazing if you neglect these key lifestyle components: stress management, sleep, and exercise. The changes I've made in these areas of my life in the past three or four years are probably *the* most profound, as I prioritize my health and enjoyment of the sweetness in life as much as I can. It's all about finding balance: I'm still ambitious enough to want to keep my businesses growing, but I

don't let it consume me the way it did when I was launching my career. I know my time with Jade is limited as she nears the end of her high school years, and I want to use these days to build memories she can share with her own family. And silly as it might sound, bringing animals into my life has also taught me invaluable lessons that I have incorporated into my daily routine. Who says you can't teach an old dog new tricks?

STRESS ◆ Stress is an unavoidable part of modern life in this country, and telling someone to avoid stress is like telling them to calm down—it inevitably has the opposite effect! I doubt we'll ever adopt the European model, where life shuts down for lunch and a siesta; here we are more likely to eat at our desk and work right through meals.

But there are steps we can take to mitigate the stress factors in our lives, especially outside office hours. One thing I've stopped doing is overscheduling. Maybe it was FOMO, maybe it was parental guilt, but I used to feel like there was something wrong if I didn't have school obligations for Jade, social engagements, or after-hours business meetings at least five nights a week. Now I try to keep business to business hours, take on only a few school projects a year, and catch up with friends via text or phone rather than hit a restaurant every time.

With a few extra hours to myself, I am able to do more of the things that help me quiet my mind and push aside the concerns of the day. Cooking a nice but uncomplicated meal, wrestling with the dogs, seeing what's going on in my herb garden, having a quiet conversation with Jade or my partner, Shane, all help me put my problems in perspective, and make me aware of how much more is right in my life than not!

Another small shift I've made is moving up my daily timeline. I used to have dinner at 8 P.M. or even later, and then go to bed directly afterward with a full stomach. Here again, I've learned from my animals. I notice that once the sun has set, they start to settle down for the night. I follow their lead and serve dinner closer to 6 P.M. these days (no cracks about the early bird special, please!). That way I can take the dogs out for a walk after dinner and get in a little movement before the end of the day but still get to bed at a reasonable hour.

My nightly routine signals the start of my serious wind down, and it's alone time that I really value. I stretch, use my foam roller to get out some kinks, and take a shower, because the hot water relaxes me. That way I'm not taking the stress of the day to bed with me. Which brings me to . . .

SLEEP ◆ I can't state this too plainly: Sleep is *vital* to good health. And as a culture we just don't value it highly enough. Sleep is when our body repairs and restores itself, and by depriving it of the time it needs to heal, we prevent the incredible machine that is our physique from operating at its highest level. If I don't get enough sleep I can't think straight, I'm foggy, and everything feels like an effort.

I used to regard sleep as the thing I did when there was nothing else more important that needed taking care of, literally the last priority on the never-ending to-do list that occupied my brain. Now I'm taking a cue from my grandfather, who used to take a nap every afternoon of his life, no matter what he was doing. I'm still not much of a napper, but unless there is a really good reason, I'm in bed by 9 every night. Once in bed, I do quiet things, like listening to an audiobook or a podcast. My favorites are memoirs—Barbra Streisand's was a recent favorite—and soothing story lines, nothing too challenging or disturbing. I try to avoid watching TV or scrolling on my phone. By 10 P.M. I'm usually drifting off to sleep, and feeling fully refreshed when I'm up at 6 the following morning to feed the animals as they start their day.

EXERCISE ◆ Here's another area in which Europeans have a radically different take from Americans. There really is not much of a gym culture there; exercise is just something that happens naturally throughout the course of the day. Movement is part of La Dolce Vita: Italians don't Uber Eats their caffeine fix, they walk out to get a coffee; and they stroll to the market every day to decide what to make for dinner. That kind of constant motion is baked into the culture. Here I can't do exactly the same thing when I'm at home in California, where everything is so spread out, but whenever possible I stand when I could be sitting and I try to walk everywhere I can. (Part of why I love spending time in NYC is that it is so walkable!)

Beyond that I do yoga four to five times a week, a hybrid form that involves a lot of stretching and mat work with light weights to work the core and develop strength without using any gym equipment or a reformer machine.

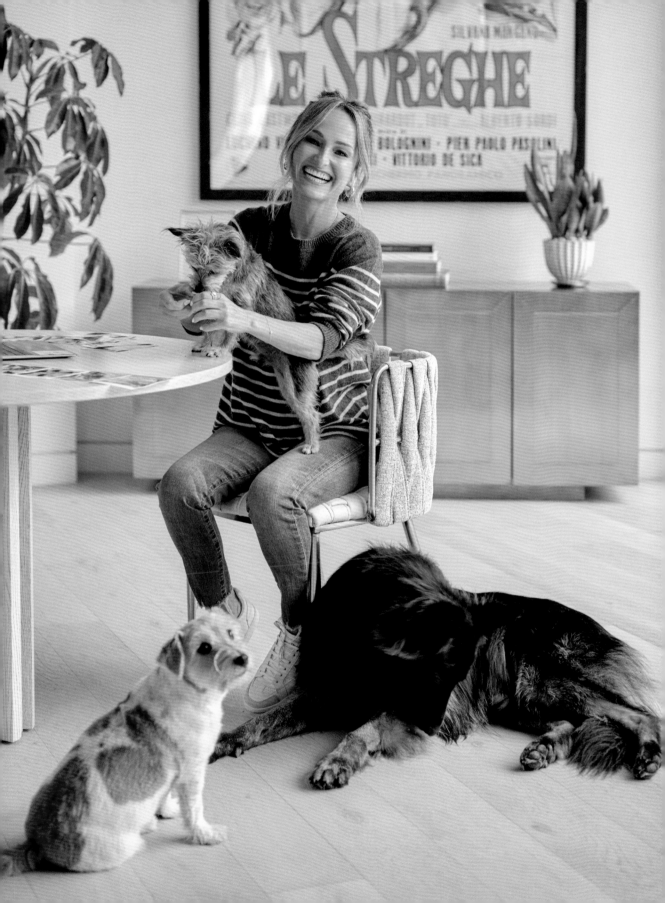

Genetics

Of all the factors that impact our health and longevity, genetics is the one that we can't really alter; we need to play the hand we are dealt. But that doesn't entirely mean that genetics are destiny. Knowing that your family is prone to diabetes or that heart disease might be a problem means that you can take steps to shore up your defenses against those conditions. And not someday, right now.

In many ways I feel I have been pretty lucky in the genetics sweepstakes. Outwardly, I take after my mother, who objectively looks and moves like a woman twenty years younger. But while I might look a certain way on the outside, on the inside there is a lot going on that isn't so pretty all the time. And with a sibling who died of cancer at a tragically young age, I know I have to be vigilant about screenings and prevention.

At the advice of my functional medicine doctor, I took a biomarker analysis test. This was an extensive panel of blood work, DNA studies, and urinalysis that looked for signs of oxidative stress, toxic exposure, mitochondrial dysfunction, and more. That's when I found out that I was a poor detoxifier and that I didn't absorb some nutrients as well as I should, indicated by moderately high levels of inflammation and oxidative stress. In layman's terms, I don't bounce back from exercise well.

We need to play the hand we are dealt. But that doesn't entirely mean that genetics are destiny.

I also had a full-body MRI that thankfully didn't reveal any abnormalities or brain atrophy (phew!). The only thing that turned up was excessive fluid in my sinuses—not terribly surprising given how prone I am to sinus infections.

I hasten to add that I recognize these tests are expensive and not usually covered by insurance, so not everyone will be able to go down this path. But I am very curious about my health and I want to be an active, not a passive, participant in my own wellness. At the end of the day, it was nice to know my organs are free of disease, but a lot of what I learned was stuff I already knew in my gut without having articulated it in so many words. I've always felt, for example, that my body takes a long time to recover from intense exercise; now I know that's because it causes oxidative stress just like an environmental toxin might! So, for me, a gentle walk with my dogs is much better than a half hour pounding away on the treadmill—it's literally in my DNA!

And now I have a baseline for comparison if something does crop up at a later date.

THESE DAYS I AM trying to learn to make peace with some of the health issues I deal with. In the past, I was always in a rush to treat every minor symptom or discomfort, sure there was a treatment, supplement, or medicine out there that would address any problem, large or small. A tiny rash would send me running to the dermatologist; a bad head cold had me wondering if I needed antibiotics. And I was taking so many supplements that I often didn't even have an appetite, all in an effort to quash

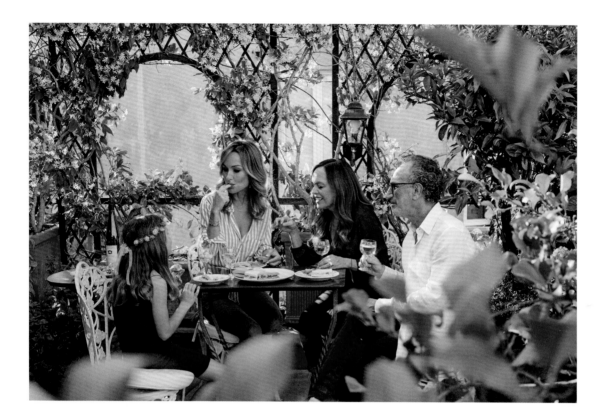

symptoms of nutritional deficiencies and forestall illnesses I didn't even have yet!

Now I'm working with a holistic doctor whose approach is less about suppressing symptoms and more about managing them and putting my body back into equilibrium. I'm trying to get more comfortable living with things, letting my body do what it needs to do before I take the nuclear option of medicating things away.

The journey of this book is finding the balance between feeling good and taking care of myself while still enjoying my life. If you spend all your emotional energy fearing the future, it's really hard to enjoy the present. And sometimes those momentary joys are worth the inevitable aftermath. Case in point: I know sugar isn't good for me, that it causes inflammation, but I have a sweet tooth that won't be denied. At this stage of my life I'm willing to put up with the inevitable discomfort that comes from overindulgence now and then, because those pleasures are at the heart of La Dolce Vita.

I guess all of this is my way of saying we all need to find our own sweet spots between indulgence and prudence, between our hearts and our heads. What works for me is not necessarily what will work for you. It's a process of trial and error. Take a look at some of the assumptions you've been living with about food, lifestyle, and priorities. Do they still serve you well? Do you make time for the things that nourish all parts of you? Are there things you can let go of in order to let more joyful experiences into your life? If so, maybe there is a pivot awaiting you, too. After all, you don't have to be Italian to benefit from the Super-Italian approach to life. Just reach out and grab the sweetness.

Now, into the kitchen!

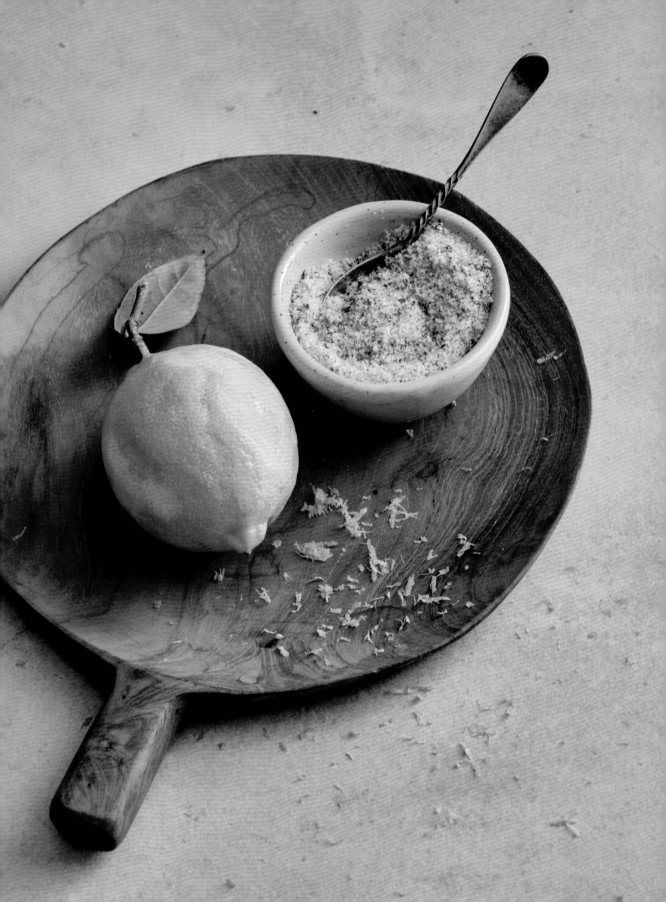

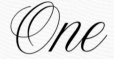

One

FLAVOR STARTS HERE:

My Essential Condiments & Basics

If there is one chapter
IN THIS BOOK

I am eager for you to dig in to, it is without a doubt this one.

These multipurpose condiments are the easiest way I know to infuse a dish with Super-Italian flavor and nutrients, and they streamline the process of making so many recipes in this book. They are also great to mix and match for dishes that taste complex but are as easy to make as ABC. Plus, they are addictively delicious.

Each one of these seasonings and sauces adds layers of flavor to food, giving the kind of depth and dimensionality you can usually only get from long, slow cook times, or complicated, chef-y methods. When you have that kind of instant flavor available by the tablespoon, splash, or dollop, cooking and preparing so many of the recipes in this book really *is* as easy as ordering in! In fact, I would even go so far as to say that armed with a few of these handy condiments, you won't even need a recipe to get a meal on the table with very little fuss or prep work.

You'll see these condiments used in every single chapter—even desserts—because they deliver intense flavor and a dash of sophistication to everything you cook. So, before you even turn to the later chapters, set aside a little time to outfit yourself with three or four of the recipes you'll find here. None of them take long to make, and all but a few will keep for weeks or longer in the fridge or freezer. Start with a big batch of seasoned salt and maybe some garlicky bread crumbs, plus a dressing like the creamy Parmesan or salsa verde and a pot of tomato sauce. You'll be amazed at how versatile they are when it comes to elevating a simple grilled meat, steamed veggie, or piece of fish into something that seems intentional. Before you know it, you will be relying on these staples to fuel your culinary improvisations and amp up their health quotients just the way I do.

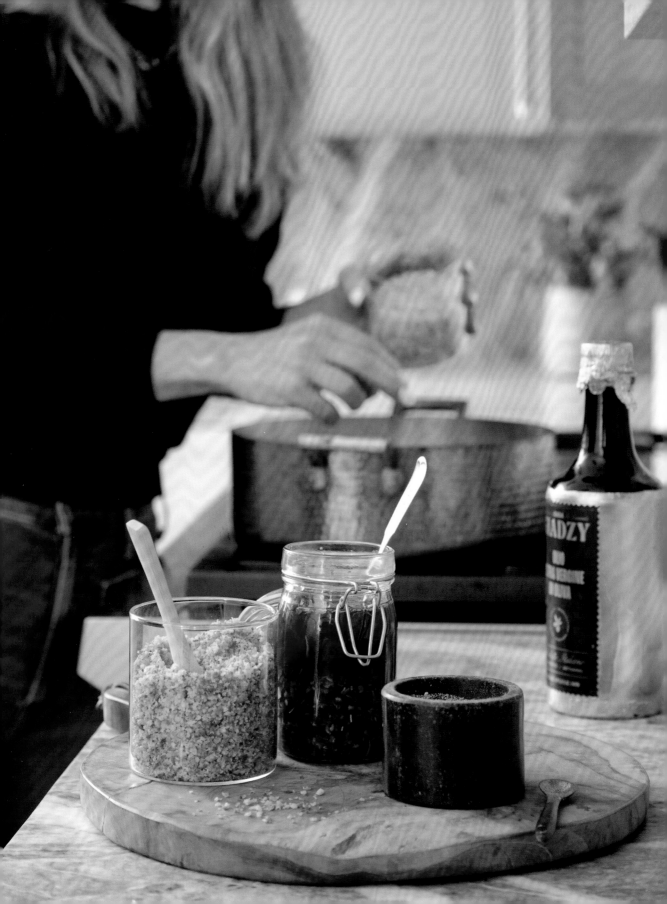

Garlicky Bread Crumbs

A better name for these might be fairy dust, because sprinkling a pinch or two on virtually anything just makes it sing. I shower them on soups, salads, and pastas when I want to add some crunch and a bit of oomph in the flavor department, but they are great on any kind of baked dish, from gratins to fish fillets, and they make an outstanding breading or stuffing. Once you've got a batch on hand, see if you don't find yourself reaching for the jar daily. They are just that good.

Makes
ABOUT 2 CUPS

3 tablespoons extra-virgin olive oil

4 large garlic cloves, smashed and peeled

¼ teaspoon red pepper flakes

4 anchovy fillets

2 cups panko bread crumbs

Grated zest of 2 small lemons

½ teaspoon kosher salt

In a medium skillet, heat the oil and garlic together over medium heat, stirring until the garlic is golden brown, 3 to 4 minutes. Use a heatproof spatula to press down on the garlic for another minute, then discard the garlic.

Add the pepper flakes and anchovies to the pan and cook with the oil, mashing with the spatula until the anchovies are completely melted into the oil. Add the panko and cook, stirring occasionally and then more frequently, until the crumbs are golden brown, about 5 minutes. Remove from the heat and stir in the lemon zest and salt.

Transfer to a plate or bowl to cool completely, then transfer to a jar with a tight-fitting lid. The crumbs can be stored at room temperature for up to 2 weeks.

USES → Breading, stuffing, finishing touch for salads and pastas, topping for gratins and baked pastas, binder in meatballs or seafood cakes.

GDL Seasoned Salt

You will find jars of sea salt blended with dried herbs and other flavorings in many Italian groceries, and they are a convenient way to add a pinch of *sapore d'Italia* (the flavor of Italy) to just about anything. The ingredients vary from region to region, with hearty winter herbs like sage and rosemary being more typical of Northern regions. I lean in a more southerly direction with my preferred mix: lemon zest, lots of Sicilian oregano, and a hint of red pepper flakes in lieu of black pepper. I never grew up eating black pepper and still don't; we always used red pepper flakes to enhance flavor. However, if you don't feel that a dish is "done" without salt and black pepper, feel free to substitute it for—or add it to—the pepper flakes. And if you have sensitive palates to feed, go ahead and leave the red pepper out altogether (or make a kid-friendly version). After all, it's *your* all-purpose seasoning, too!

Makes
1 CUP

3 to 4 teaspoons red pepper flakes (preferably Calabrian)

2 tablespoons dried Sicilian oregano

1 teaspoon dried rosemary

1 cup kosher salt

2 lemons

With a mortar and pestle, coffee/spice grinder, or small blender, briefly blitz the red pepper flakes, oregano, and rosemary to a coarse powder; you want to see small bits, not just dust. Set aside.

Place the salt in a small bowl. Using a Microplane, grate the zest of the lemons directly into the bowl, capturing all the fragrant oil from the peel as well as the zest. (Reserve the lemons for another use.) Use your fingertips to rub the zest into the salt.

Add the pulverized red pepper flake/herb mixture to the bowl and combine. Transfer to a jar with a tight-fitting lid. The salt will be good indefinitely, but the flavors will lose potency over time.

USES ◆ Popcorn, steamed veggies, focaccia, breading, eggs—basically anything!

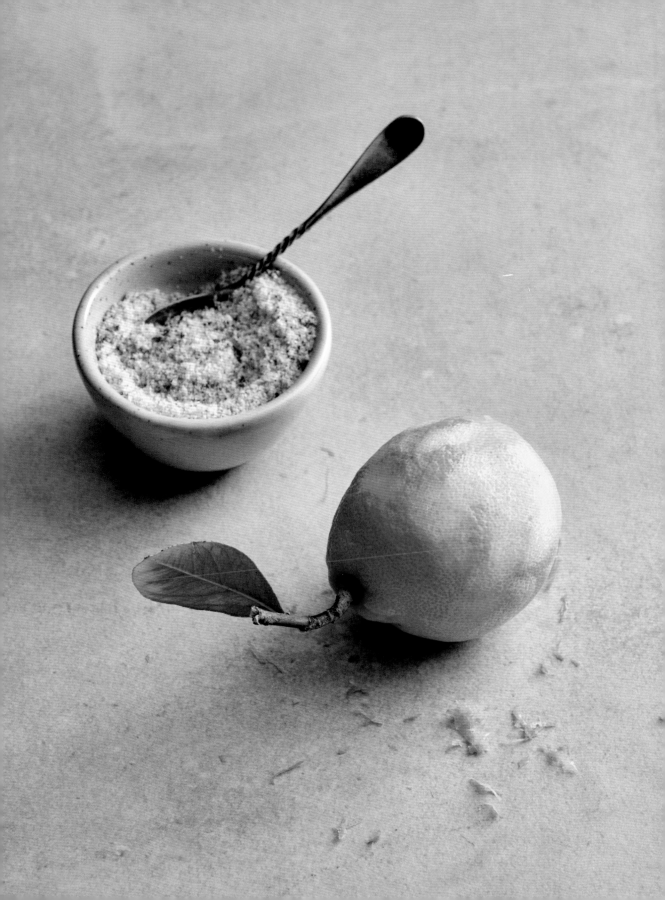

Calabrian Chile Garlic Oil

If you like Asian chili crisp, I'm willing to bet you will *love* this crunchy topper, with just the right amount of heat, a subtle hint of sweetness, and loads of umami thanks to the mushroom powder. Spoon it on your avocado toast or a Caprese salad to give those old standards new life, or just set it out on the table and let everyone add a dab to their pasta, seafood, or veggies. The most important step is cooking the shallots and garlic *just* until golden; don't rush it, stir often, and keep an eye on it, because if it gets too dark (or the garlic burns), the whole batch goes down the drain.

Makes
ABOUT 1½ CUPS

3 tablespoons red pepper flakes (preferably Calabrian)

2 teaspoons kosher salt

1 teaspoon sugar

1 tablespoon dried Sicilian oregano, crumbled

1 teaspoon dried rosemary, crumbled

1½ teaspoons porcini mushroom powder (see Hint)

1 cup extra-virgin olive oil

3 shallots, finely chopped (about ½ cup)

6 garlic cloves, finely chopped (about ¼ cup)

½ teaspoon colatura

In a heatproof glass measuring cup, combine the pepper flakes, salt, sugar, oregano, rosemary, and mushroom powder. Set a sieve on top and set aside.

In a saucepan, combine the oil and shallots. Bring to a simmer over medium-high heat, then adjust the heat so the shallots bubble gently. Continue to cook the shallots, stirring often, until the majority are light golden brown, about 8 minutes. The bits around the edges will color first, so keep stirring to distribute the darker bits while the rest cook.

When about three-quarters of the shallots are golden (but no darker), add the garlic. Cook, stirring, until everything is golden, about 90 seconds.

Immediately remove the pan from the heat and pour the hot oil through the sieve onto the pepper flakes and herbs. Stir the oil to combine and let the fried shallots and garlic cool completely. When cooled, stir the fried bits into the flavored oil. Stir in the colatura and transfer to a jar with a lid. The condiment will last for a month or more in the refrigerator.

HINT HINT ◆ Porcini powder is available online, but it is easy to make your own. Just place a handful of dried porcini mushrooms in a coffee grinder, spice grinder, or small blender. Whiz until the mushrooms are pulverized to a fine powder. The powder will keep indefinitely but the flavor and aroma will diminish over time.

USES ◆ Eggs, avocado toast, dips, stir-fries, noodle dishes, seafood.

Do-It-All Parmesan Dressing

With a gorgeous pale green color, savory Parmesan top note, and slightly sweet aftertaste, this is so much more than a salad dressing. It works as a dip for crudités and fried seafood, would be great in a wrap sandwich, and is delicious on steamed vegetables or in a potato salad. And on a salad? It will have even staunch salad skeptics licking their plates. Go ahead and make a double batch; you'll be glad you did.

Makes
ABOUT 1½ CUPS

⅔ cup extra-virgin olive oil

¼ cup fresh lemon juice
(about 2 large lemons)

2 tablespoons apple cider vinegar

1 tablespoon honey

2 teaspoons Dijon mustard

1½ teaspoons kosher salt

1 cup freshly grated
Parmigiano-Reggiano cheese

8 large fresh basil leaves

2 garlic cloves,
smashed and peeled

In a small blender (see Hint), combine the oil, lemon juice, vinegar, honey, mustard, salt, cheese, and basil and blend until smooth and well emulsified. Transfer the dressing to a storage jar and add the garlic. Cover and refrigerate, allowing the garlic to gently infuse the dressing until you are ready to use it. Store in the refrigerator for up to 1 week, discarding the garlic after a day or two.

HINT HINT ◆ You can also make this with an immersion blender or in a food processor, but it won't be quite as green or creamy. The blender whips in a bit more air, which changes the texture. Either way it will taste delicious.

USES ◆ Salads, raw veggies, sandwiches, grilled or sautéed white fish.

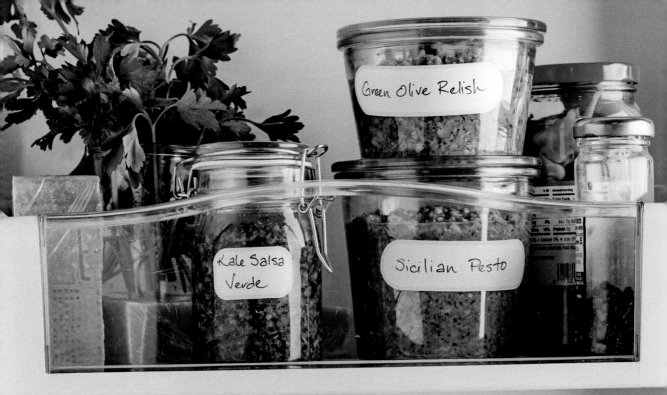

Green Olive Relish

Kale Salsa Verde

Sicilian Pesto

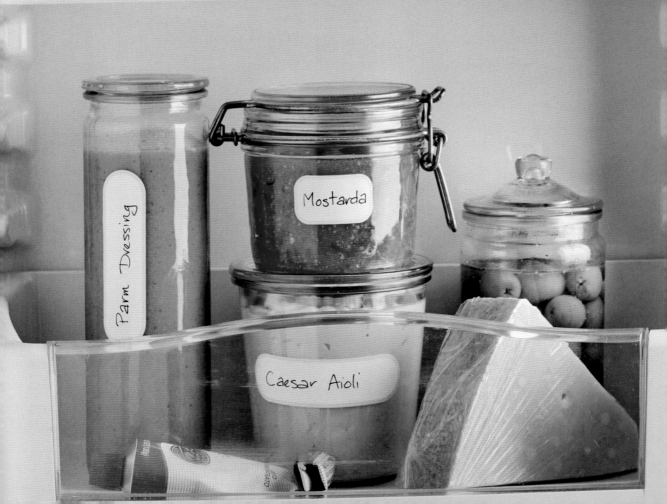

Parm Dressing

Mostarda

Caesar Aioli

Caesar Aioli

If you think mayonnaise is boring, think again; this smooth, creamy sauce can be used as a dip, dressing, sandwich spread, or topping and packs all the bright, punchy flavors of your favorite Caesar dressing. I've used colatura, Italy's version of fish sauce, to provide the anchovy kick, but if you only have anchovies on hand, just use the side of a chef's knife to mash an anchovy fillet and the salt to a paste.

Makes
A GENEROUS 1 CUP

1 large egg yolk

1 garlic clove, grated on a Microplane

1 teaspoon Dijon mustard

½ teaspoon colatura

2 tablespoons fresh lemon juice, plus more to taste

¼ teaspoon Calabrian chile paste (optional)

¾ cup neutral oil, such as canola or grapeseed

¼ cup extra-virgin olive oil

½ teaspoon kosher salt, plus more to taste

¼ cup freshly grated Parmigiano-Reggiano cheese

In a medium bowl, whisk together the egg yolk, garlic, mustard, colatura, lemon juice, and chile paste (if using) until completely smooth. Combine the oils in a measuring cup and, whisking constantly, slowly beat the oil into the egg yolk mixture. Start by adding just a drop or two at a time, increasing the flow of oil as the mixture thickens to a creamy, mayonnaise-y consistency. (See Hint.) When all the oil has been incorporated, stir in the salt and Parmigiano. Taste and add a bit more lemon juice or salt if necessary.

Store in an airtight container in the refrigerator for up to 1 week.

HINT HINT ◆ It is important to add the oil bit by bit when making this by hand, but if you use an immersion blender you can add all the oil at once. Plunge the blender to the bottom of your mixing vessel and blend, pulling up the wand slowly (rather than plunging it up and down) until thick.

USES ◆ Salad dressings, sandwiches, hot or room-temperature steamed vegetables, egg salad or deviled eggs, fish soups or stews, dip for crudités or steamed artichokes, dressing for potato or pasta salads.

Kale Salsa Verde

If you're looking for an easy way to infuse some Super-Italian energy into your cooking, look no further than this tangy green condiment, which is made of nothing *but* superfoods! Every bite delivers a vibrant hit of herbs, capers, olives, and citrus, with all the goodness of Tuscan kale (and a touch of anchovy, for depth and salty flavor). Its brightness is especially good with fish and seafood, and it cuts through the fatty flavor of grilled or roasted meats beautifully.

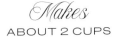

Makes
ABOUT 2 CUPS

◆

1 small shallot, roughly chopped

1 garlic clove, roughly chopped

1 cup curly or lacinato (Tuscan) kale, stripped off the center rib

2 tablespoons (packed) fresh mint leaves

2 tablespoons (packed) fresh flat-leaf Italian parsley

10 fresh chives

2 tablespoons drained capers

3 anchovy fillets

8 Cerignola or Castelvetrano olives, pitted

Grated zest and juice of 1 lemon

½ teaspoon Calabrian chile paste

½ teaspoon kosher salt

1 cup extra-virgin olive oil

In a food processor or blender, combine all the ingredients and pulse on and off until the kale and herbs are finely chopped but not pureed. Transfer to a jar and store in the refrigerator for up to 2 weeks. Allow the salsa verde to return to room temperature and then stir or shake well before serving.

USES ◆ Grilled meats, salad dressing, dip, tuna or egg salad, garnish for bean soups or risottos.

Green Olive Relish

At first glance this might appear similar to Kale Salsa Verde [page 54], but the orange juice and zest make this a sweeter, milder, brighter alternative that is lovely with mild fish or vegetables. Try it on a cheese platter or as a topping for crostini, too. You can make it entirely in the food processor if you prefer, but don't overprocess it; you want some chunky texture, not a smooth puree. I've used fresh oregano here because it is the herb of choice in many olive-growing regions, but if you don't have any on hand, parsley, basil, mint, even cilantro would all be delicious alternatives.

Makes
ABOUT 1 CUP

1 small shallot

1 cup pitted Castelvetrano olives

1 tablespoon drained capers

1 small garlic clove, peeled

Grated zest and juice of 1 orange

2 tablespoons extra-virgin olive oil

2 tablespoons red wine vinegar

1 tablespoon chopped fresh oregano

½ teaspoon kosher salt

Thinly slice the shallot, place in a small bowl with water to cover, and soak for 15 minutes. Drain well and transfer to a food processor.

Add the olives and capers and pulse just until finely minced but not pureed to a paste. Transfer to a bowl. Use a Microplane to grate the garlic directly into the bowl. Add the orange zest, orange juice, oil, vinegar, oregano, and salt and stir to combine. Store the relish in an airtight container in the refrigerator for up to 2 weeks.

USES ◆ Cutlets or grilled fish, pastas, grain or pasta salads, salad dressings.

Parmesan Basil Butter

The beauty of flavored butters like this one is that they are at their best when made ahead so you have them at your disposal to add to veggies, fish, potatoes, or rice at any time. I like to store mine in the freezer and grate them, because the little bits incorporate so easily. If you prefer to use it by the slice, you can refrigerate it or transfer it from the freezer to the fridge the night before you plan to use it. Make this at the height of summer, when luxuriant bunches of basil arrive in the farmers' market, because you need a generous amount of basil for it, and the overpriced hydroponic stems available in winter rarely have enough flavor. Then store it in the freezer to add a dash of summery freshness to dishes all year long.

Makes
1 CUP

1 cup (packed) fresh basil leaves

1 small garlic clove, peeled

2 sticks (8 ounces) unsalted butter, cut into chunks, at room temperature

¾ cup freshly grated Parmigiano-Reggiano cheese

½ teaspoon kosher salt

Fill a large bowl with water and ice and set it near your sink. Bring a large pot of salted water to a boil. Add the basil and blanch for 15 to 20 seconds, stirring to ensure all the leaves are submerged. Immediately drain the basil and dump into the ice bath, swishing the leaves to separate and cool quickly. Drain the leaves again, gently pressing to squeeze out as much water as possible.

Transfer the basil to a food processor and pulse until very finely chopped. Grate the garlic on a Microplane directly into the processor bowl. Add the butter. Pulse on and off until the butter is creamy and uniformly green, scraping it down from time to time and spreading it out if it forms a clump. Add the cheese and salt and pulse to combine.

Scrape half the butter onto each of two sheets of parchment. Lift the paper and drop it on the counter once or twice to release some of the air that was beaten into the butter, then use a spatula to shape it into a log. Roll the butter tightly, twisting the ends of the paper to seal. Refrigerate for up to 2 weeks or freeze for 3 months or longer. It's a good idea to store the wrapped logs in a heavy freezer bag if you plan to keep them frozen longer than a couple of weeks to prevent freezer burn and protect the butter from picking up other flavors.

USES ◆ Steamed or sautéed vegetables; popcorn; rice, pasta, or potatoes; roast chicken (under the skin); pan sauces; scrambled eggs; toast or ham sandwich.

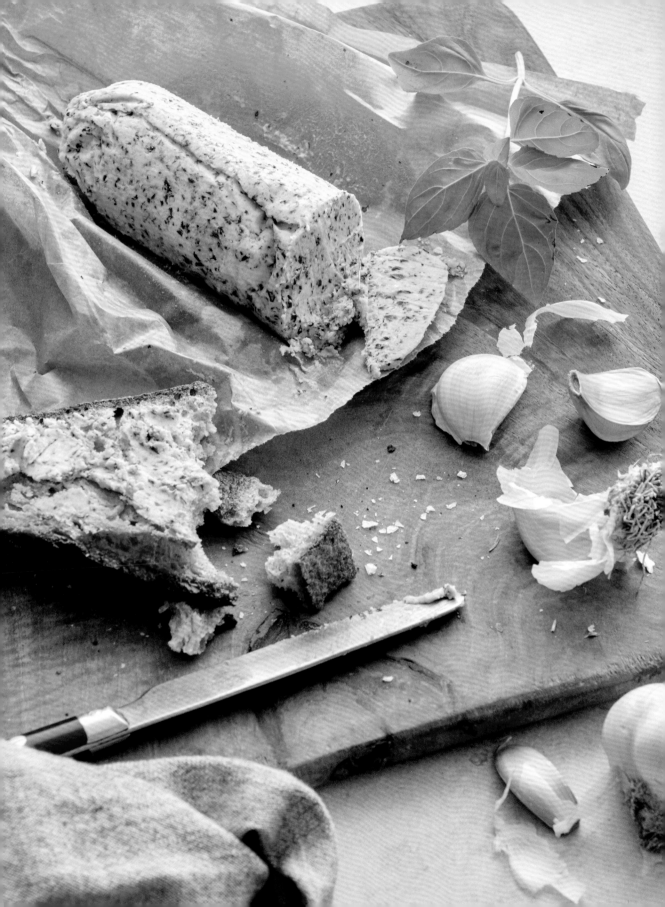

Summer Mostarda

Somewhere between a jam and a chutney, with a tangy, spicy bite, this sweet-and-savory condiment is especially good with poultry and pork, or with creamy foods like cheese. Make the chunks large or small, as you prefer. If peaches are not in season, you can easily use frozen, reducing the cooking time by a minute or two, or substitute another fruit like pears, plums, or apples and omit the tomato.

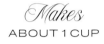

Makes
ABOUT 1 CUP

1 tablespoon extra-virgin olive oil

1 small shallot, diced

1 large peach or 1½ cups frozen peaches, cut into ¾-inch pieces

1 large plum tomato, cut into ¾-inch pieces

¼ cup apple cider vinegar

3 tablespoons sugar

1 tablespoon mustard seeds

2 teaspoons mustard powder

¼ teaspoon kosher salt

1 teaspoon Calabrian chile paste

1 fresh rosemary sprig

In a saucepan, heat the oil over medium heat. Add the shallot and sauté for 2 or 3 minutes to soften; don't allow it to brown. Add the peach, tomato, vinegar, sugar, mustard seeds, mustard powder, salt, chile paste, and rosemary. Add ¼ cup water to the pan and stir to combine.

Bring the mixture to a simmer and cook over medium-low heat until the fruit is softened but still chunky and the liquid is somewhat thickened, about 10 minutes. Use a heatproof spatula to stir frequently, especially as it thickens, to prevent it from scorching, and add a bit more water to the pan if it starts to seem too dry.

Cool slightly, then transfer to a jar. The mostarda can be stored in the refrigerator for up to 2 weeks.

USES ◆ Charcuterie plate, cheese sandwiches, roast meat, salad dressing (chopped finely).

Peperonata

My family often made this tangy blend of peppers and olives in extra-large batches to serve in different guises over the course of a week. The first night it would be served warm as a side dish with meat or fish, the next night we might toss some with pasta, and later on it might turn up as part of a cold antipasto spread or on a sandwich—you get the idea. It's the perfect way to salvage a bell pepper or two you've forgotten in the crisper drawer, and once you get in the habit of having this versatile relish on hand, I think you'll find your own ways to use it throughout the week.

Makes
ABOUT 2 CUPS

2 tablespoons extra-virgin olive oil

3 garlic cloves, smashed and peeled

2 anchovy fillets

1 small red onion, halved and thinly sliced

2 large bell peppers, preferably one red and one yellow, thinly sliced

¾ teaspoon kosher salt

¼ cup chopped kalamata olives

2 tablespoons balsamic vinegar

1 tablespoon drained capers

1 teaspoon chopped fresh oregano

In a medium skillet, heat the oil over medium heat. Add the garlic and anchovies and cook, breaking up the anchovies with a wooden spoon, until the garlic is golden and the anchovies have melted into the oil, about 2 minutes. Add the onion and cook, stirring, until starting to soften, about 2 minutes. Add the peppers and salt and cook until the onions are caramelized and the peppers are starting to brown, 8 to 10 minutes.

Remove from the heat and stir in the olives, vinegar, capers, and oregano. Serve warm, cold, or at room temperature.

USES ◆ Side dish, simple pasta sauce, baked or sautéed seafood, stuffing for baked vegetables, antipasto spread.

Sicilian Pesto

In the United States, the term "pesto" has become synonymous with the Genovese basil-and-pignoli paste that became popular here in the '70s. Traveling through Italy, though, you will quickly come to realize that pesto looks and tastes different from region to region and refers to a wide and delicious variety of herby pastes, all made with the ingredients that are most plentiful locally. I'm obsessed with this pale orange version from the South of Italy. The bright astringency of cherry tomatoes and nutty flavor of almonds make it a sweeter, brighter pesto than what you're probably accustomed to, and it's such a great complement to seafood, cheese, and pasta.

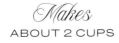

Makes
ABOUT 2 CUPS

½ cup slivered almonds

1 pint cherry tomatoes

1 cup (lightly packed) fresh basil leaves

1 garlic clove, roughly chopped

1½ teaspoons kosher salt

½ teaspoon red pepper flakes

½ cup extra-virgin olive oil

¾ cup freshly grated Parmigiano-Reggiano cheese

In a dry skillet, toast the almonds over medium heat just until fragrant and very lightly golden, 3 to 4 minutes. Spread on a plate to cool for a few minutes, then transfer to a food processor.

Add the tomatoes, basil, garlic, salt, and pepper flakes to the food processor and pulse until finely chopped. With the machine running, slowly stream in the oil. Add the cheese and pulse once or twice to combine.

Store the pesto in a jar with a tight-fitting lid in the refrigerator for up to 2 weeks.

USES ◆ Pastas and pasta salads, dip for crudités or seafood, steamed vegetables, crostini.

Calabrian Pomodoro

When I want a heartier, more robust sauce than my Simple Tomato Sauce [page 63], with just a bit of heat, this is the one I reach for. It's chunkier, with a more traditional flavor thanks to the oregano; and although it only cooks for about 20 minutes in total, it tastes rich and well rounded. I always make it with imported canned cherry tomatoes because I find them sweeter, more flavorful, and less acidic than canned plum tomatoes. If you don't love spice, or are cooking for little ones, leave out the chile paste or use Simple Tomato Sauce instead.

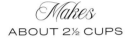

Makes
ABOUT 2½ CUPS

¼ cup extra-virgin olive oil

2 (14-ounce) cans Italian cherry tomatoes, undrained

1 to 2 teaspoons Calabrian chile paste

1 teaspoon dried oregano

4 teaspoons kosher salt, plus more to taste

2 teaspoons grated lemon zest

2 teaspoons fresh lemon juice

2 tablespoons unsalted butter

In a medium saucepan, heat the oil over medium heat. Add the tomatoes and their juices, crushing the tomatoes a bit with your hands as you add them to the pot. Rinse out the cans with ¼ cup water and add that to the pot as well. Add the chile paste, oregano, salt, and lemon zest and juice and bring to a simmer over medium heat. Reduce the heat to low and cook at a gentle simmer for 10 minutes, stirring occasionally and crushing the tomatoes against the side of the pan.

Add the butter and stir to incorporate. Taste and season with a bit more salt if needed. Store in a container with a tight-fitting lid in the fridge for up to 5 days; freeze for up to 3 months.

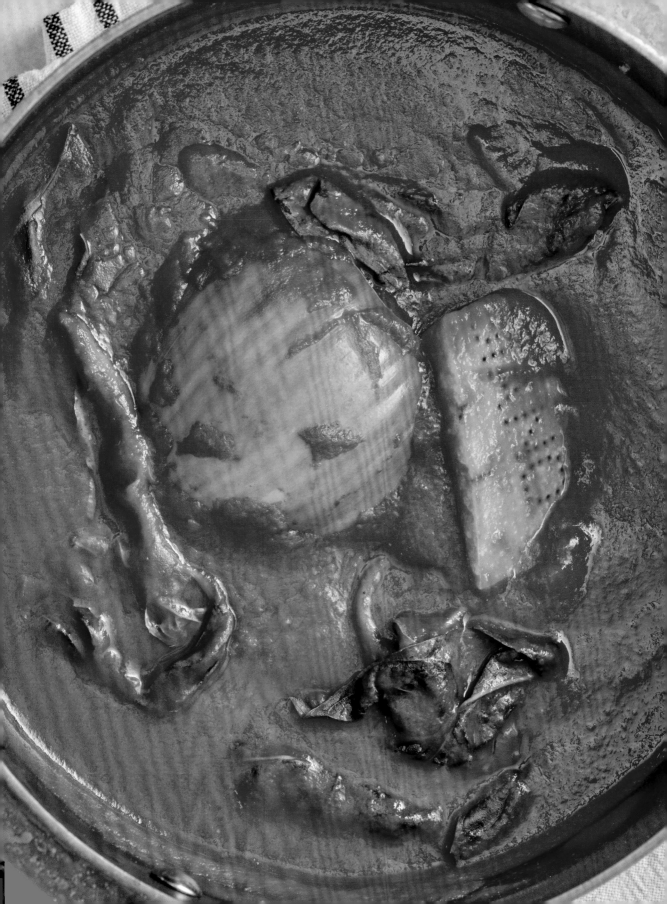

Simple Tomato Sauce

My family made this quick, smooth sauce on repeat, preparing a double or even triple batch at least once a week. I recommend you do the same, because it is an excellent, all-purpose sauce that works in many different dishes. Because it is made with passata—tomatoes that have simply been pureed and strained—it has a bright, fresh flavor you don't get from long-cooked sauces, and a bit of richness from the Parm rinds and a teeny bit of butter. Seek out a good imported brand of passata in a jar if you can.

Makes
ABOUT 3 CUPS

1 (24-ounce) jar passata
(tomato puree)

½ red onion

1 to 3 garlic cloves, to taste

5 stalks fresh basil

2-inch piece
Parmigiano-Reggiano rind

¾ teaspoon kosher salt

1 to 2 tablespoons unsalted butter,
to taste

Pour the passata into a medium saucepan. Rinse the jar out with ¼ cup water and add to the pan along with the onion, garlic, basil, and Parm rind. Bring to a simmer over medium heat, then reduce the heat to low, partially cover, and simmer for 20 minutes.

Discard the solids. Add the salt, then stir in the butter until melted. Store in a jar with a tight-fitting lid in the refrigerator and use within 5 days. Freeze extras for up to 3 months.

Parmesan Chicken Broth

Good strong chicken broth is the backbone of so many recipes and not just soups and risottos; you'll find it adds flavor to all kinds of vegetable and grain dishes—even pasta sauces! I fortify mine with the essence of Parmesan by simmering some chunks of rind along with the chicken. Many supermarkets that sell grated cheese in their deli section now package up the rinds (or give them away if you ask nicely!), so stock up whenever you see them. They can be frozen indefinitely. I don't salt the stock as I find the Parm adds enough salty flavor.

Makes
3 QUARTS

1 large onion, halved

3 to 4 pounds chicken pieces or two meaty carcasses (see Hint)

2 carrots, chopped

2 celery stalks, chopped

1 head garlic, halved through the equator

2 (2-inch) pieces Parmigiano-Reggiano rind

10 fresh thyme sprigs

1 bay leaf

½ teaspoon black peppercorns

Place the onion cut side down in a dry soup pot and cook over medium heat until deep golden brown, about 5 minutes. Add the chicken, carrots, celery, garlic, Parm rinds, thyme, bay leaf, and peppercorns and cover with 4 quarts of cold water. Bring to a boil over high heat, then immediately reduce the heat to low. Skim the surface with a fine sieve or a slotted spoon to remove the foam and impurities that rise to the surface. Partially cover the pot and simmer for about 2 hours, or until well flavored, skimming off any foam now and then.

Strain the broth, discarding the solids (I pick off the meat from the chicken bones and save it to mix with my dogs' food), and portion it out into storage containers. When cool, refrigerate. Fat will rise to the top and solidify, so you can skim it off either the next day or just before using. The broth can be stored in the refrigerator for up to 1 week or frozen for 3 months or longer.

HINT HINT ◆ If you are in the habit of saving the carcasses from rotisserie chickens, this is a great way to use them. Otherwise you can use raw chicken parts: Leg/thigh quarters will produce a more strongly flavored broth than breasts, so buy accordingly.

Savory Vegetable Broth

The quality and flavors of vegetable broth in a box are so variable; some taste of too much onion, some of too much celery, others are way too salty, and still others taste like nothing much at all. I like mine to be balanced and not too oniony, with a hint of sweetness from the fennel.

Makes
ABOUT 6 CUPS

◆

½ onion

2 tomatoes, halved

4 garlic cloves,
smashed and peeled

2 carrots, cut into thirds

2 celery stalks, cut into thirds

½ fennel bulb with stalks and fronds,
cut into 4 wedges

15 fresh thyme sprigs

8 stalks fresh flat-leaf Italian parsley

1 bay leaf

½ teaspoon whole black
peppercorns

Place the onion and tomatoes in a large heavy saucepan or Dutch oven over medium heat. Cook without moving until the onion is deep golden brown, about 5 minutes.

Add the garlic, carrots, celery, fennel, thyme, parsley, bay leaf, peppercorns, and 8 cups cold water to cover. Bring to a simmer over medium-high heat, partially cover, and simmer gently for 1 hour. If any foam or impurities rise to the surface, use a fine sieve or slotted spoon to skim them off and discard.

Strain the broth into storage containers, discarding the solids, and cool to room temperature. Store the broth in the refrigerator for 1 week or freeze for up to 3 months.

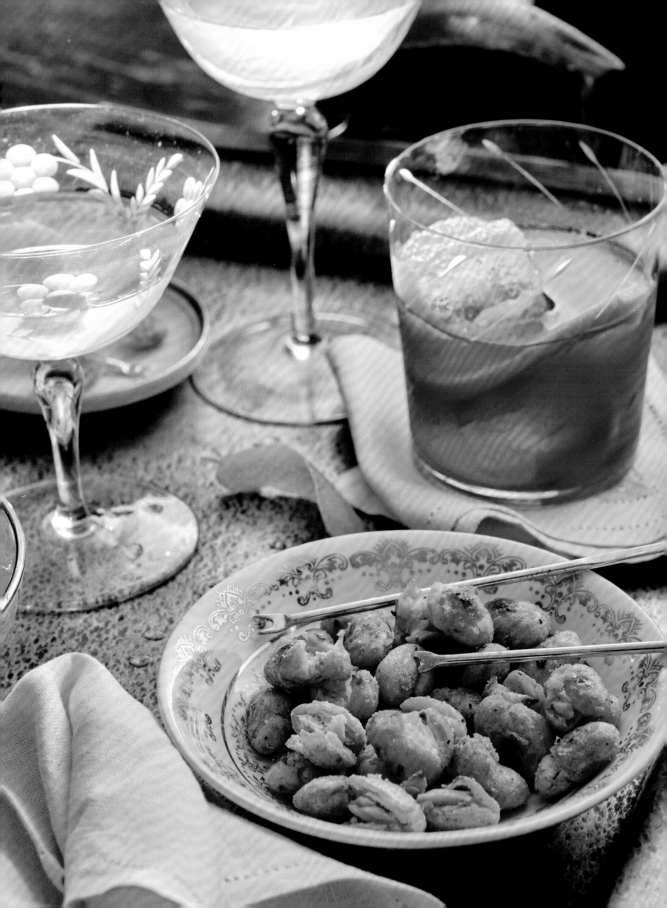

Two
—— · ——

Cocktails
& Apps

———— ◆ ————

Few things exemplify

THE ART OF LA DOLCE VITA

better than the Italian ritual of aperitivi. At the hour when most Americans are heading home to start dinner, Italians are flocking to cafés for a cocktail and some small nibbles, a way to signal that the workday is done and the transition to the evening's pleasures—dinner with friends, a gathering, an unhurried family meal—has begun.

When I entertain, I like to take my cue from this custom. Unless it's an appetizer party, I keep the offerings light and simple: just something to break the ice and whet the appetite. I always have a themed cocktail because it's a conversation starter and brings people together. It's the first thing people see and taste when they come to your home, so it should be pretty and it should be delicious. And I make sure to have plenty of nonalcoholic options available, too.

Along with the cocktails I will put out one or maybe two nibbles, elegant enough to show that I've made an effort but easy enough that they don't pull focus from the main event. It's tempting to default to a classic charcuterie platter for company, but to me, that's a heavy (not to mention calorically dense) way to start an evening. At the same time, I want people to feel super special and that's not the message sent by a bowl of chips or a handful of nuts.

Instead, I reach for the condiment cupboard, using seasoned salt to turn a dish of my best olive oil into a dip for fancy crudités, or adorning some simple crostini with a dab of fruity mostarda or a spoonful of peperonata. It's tasty, it's incredibly fast to put together, and it leaves my guests with plenty of room for the fabulous dinner awaiting them. And if they are starting off the evening with a few of my Super-Italian superfoods, I doubt any of them will be any the wiser—just healthier!

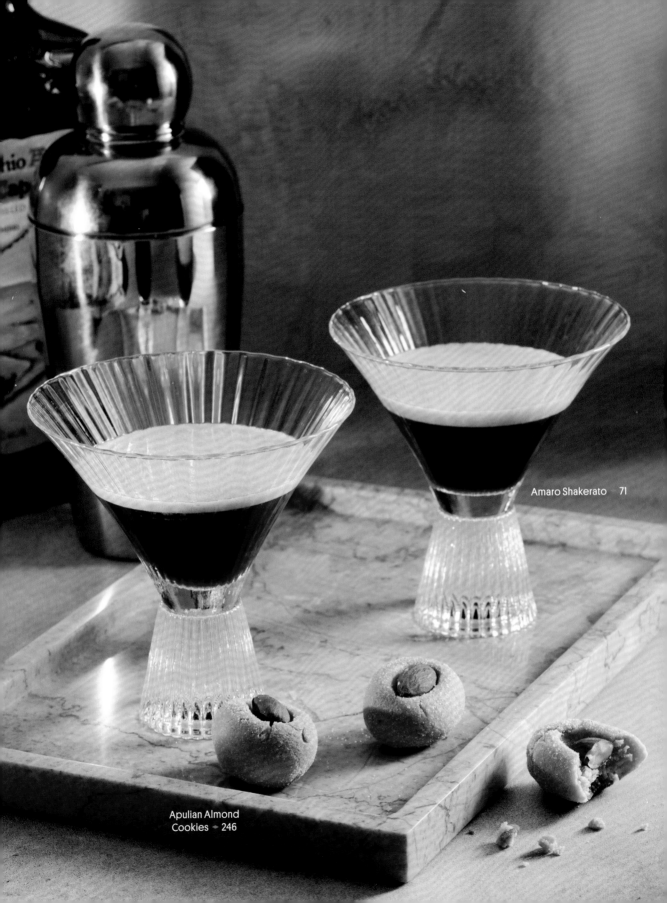

Amaro Shakerato   71

Apulian Almond
Cookies ← 246

Amaro Shakerato

Coffee shakerato, a frothy, creamy cold beverage made by shaking coffee with ice, is something I only started enjoying as an adult on trips home to Italy. When my uncle Aurelio owned a soccer team in Naples, my cousins and I would hang out in a café and catch up over shakeratos while waiting to head over to a game. I've added a hit of herbaceous amaro to the mix for a lightly boozy version that works as well after dinner as before.

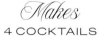

Makes
4 COCKTAILS

6 ounces amaro (I like Caffo Vecchio Amaro del Capo from Calabria)

6 ounces cold brew coffee

Combine the ingredients in a jar and refrigerate until very cold, at least 1 hour. Pour into a blender and whiz until the mixture is foamy, 10 to 15 seconds. Divide among four martini glasses and serve.

Lemon-Thyme Prosecco Cocktail

Try this pretty, fragrant cocktail when you need a less-expected alternative to an Aperol Spritz. It has a similar sweet-tart flavor with none of the bitterness and a lower alcohol content. Note that you need to prepare the lemonade ice cubes ahead of time. When I was a kid, pink lemonade was everything to me, I even dipped my Oreos in it! Now I use it to make this refreshing summer drink that I enjoy wherever in the world I find myself—Capri, the Hamptons, or here in California.

Serves
6

2 cups pink lemonade

12 fresh thyme sprigs, preferably lemon thyme

1 (750 ml) bottle prosecco, chilled

The day before serving, pour the lemonade into silicone ice cube molds. Place in the freezer and freeze until solid, at least 8 hours.

Place 2 lemonade ice cubes in each of 6 champagne flutes. Add 2 sprigs of thyme to each glass, rubbing the sprigs gently with your fingers over the glass to release their oils. Fill the glasses with prosecco and serve.

Limoncello Martini

Limoncello was huge in my house, but we mostly served it as an after-dinner drink. I like to add a dash to my martini because it adds a touch of sweetness, and holding a martini makes me feel like an old-time Hollywood movie star, elegant and timeless. Less sweet than a Lemon Drop, less potent than a dirty martini, this variation on the 50/50 martini has a subtle sweet-and-savory flavor that goes perfectly with salty nibbles, like nuts or Crunchy Roasted Butter Beans [page 81].

Makes
1 COCKTAIL

Ice

1½ ounces gin

1½ ounces dry vermouth

1 teaspoon limoncello

1 strip of lemon zest, for garnish
[see Hint]

Fill a cocktail shaker or tall glass with ice. Add the gin, vermouth, and limoncello. Use a bar spoon to stir for 20 to 30 seconds to dilute the mixture slightly, then strain into a chilled coupe or martini glass. Garnish with the lemon zest and serve.

HINT HINT ◆ For more lemon aroma, rub the rim of the glass with the lemon zest, then fold it in half lengthwise and squeeze over the cocktail to release the oil from the peel on the surface of the cocktail.

The "Mi-To"

This precursor to the Negroni is popular at the bar of my Las Vegas restaurant, and it's a perfect [if potent!] aperitif. The name, shorthand for Milano Torino, refers to the birthplace of its two components. At Giada Vegas we use authentic Vermouth di Torino, but any sweet red vermouth will work.

Makes
1 COCKTAIL

Ice

1½ ounces Campari

1½ ounces sweet red vermouth

1 orange slice, for garnish

Fill a cocktail glass with ice. Add the Campari and sweet vermouth and stir for about 10 seconds to mix and slightly dilute. Add the orange slice and serve.

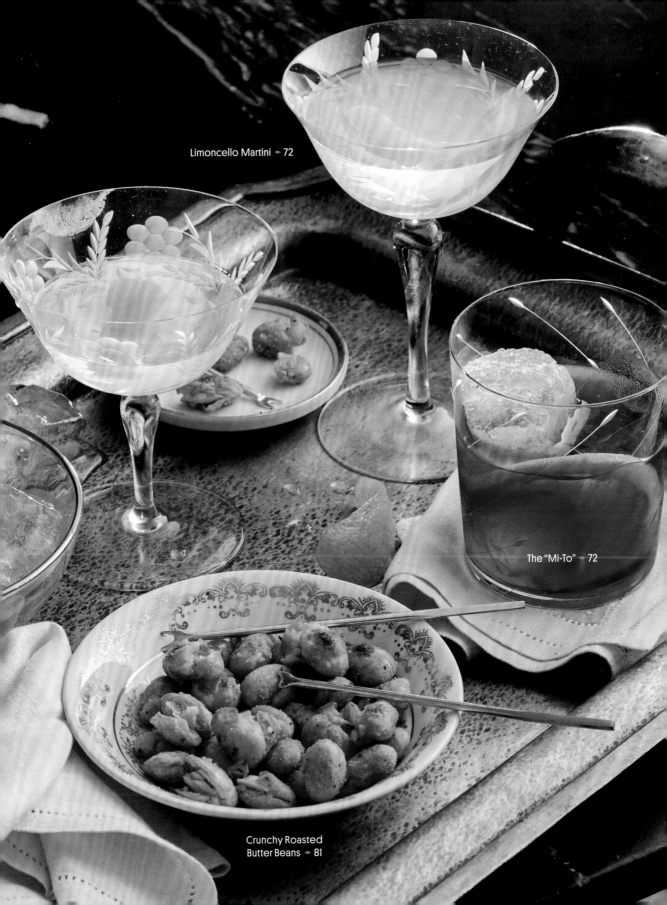

Limoncello Martini → 72

The "Mi-To" → 72

Crunchy Roasted
Butter Beans → 81

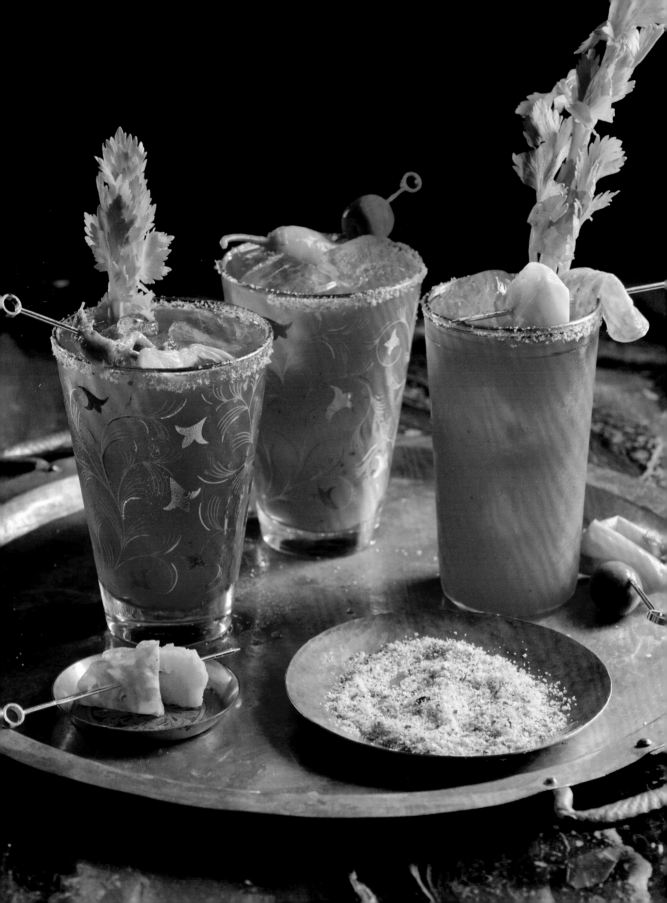

Bloody Maria

I've given this brunch staple an Italian makeover for a pitcher drink that goes perfectly with cheese, crostini, or, yes, an omelet. Have fun with the garnishes; you could spear a piece of salami, an anchovy, even a chunk of Parmigiano to nestle into each drink. If you, like me, are a fennel lover, save the tough upper stalks that usually go in the soup pot to stand in for the celery stirrer.

Serves
4 TO 6

¼ cup GDL Seasoned Salt
[page 48]

1 lemon

2½ cups tomato juice

¾ cup vodka

¼ cup brine from a jar of
pepperoncini

½ teaspoon colatura or 1 teaspoon
Worcestershire sauce

¼ teaspoon freshly ground
black pepper

Ice

8 to 12 green olives, for garnish

4 to 6 pepperoncini, for garnish

4 to 6 tender celery stalks or leafy
fennel stalks, for stirring

Place the seasoned salt on a small plate. Squeeze the lemon into a pitcher, then use the squeezed rinds to wet the rims of four to six tall glasses. Roll the rims in the seasoned salt and set aside to dry.

To the pitcher, add the tomato juice, vodka, pepperoncini brine, colatura, and pepper. Chill until ready to serve.

To serve, place a few ice cubes in each of the prepared glasses and fill with the cocktail mixture. Spear 2 olives and a pepperoncino on a toothpick and place atop the cocktail, then add a celery stalk stirrer.

Strawberry-Basil Agua Fresca

I have so many little kids in my family now that I am always on the hunt for festive drinks that everyone can enjoy. This one gives pool party punch vibes and is really hydrating on a hot summer day. Make it ahead of time, adding the last 2 cups of water just before serving in a tall glass with plenty of ice.

Serves
6 TO 8

1 pound strawberries, hulled

½ cup sugar

4 large fresh basil leaves, plus sprigs for garnish

2 tablespoons fresh lemon juice

Ice

In a blender, combine the strawberries, sugar, basil leaves, and lemon juice and puree on high speed until fairly smooth, about 1 minute. Add 2 cups cold water and puree for another minute. Pour the mixture into a large pitcher and stir in another 2 cups cold water. Garnish with additional basil sprigs.

Serve over ice.

Mushroom-Stuffed Mushrooms

This is an oldie but goodie that works equally well as a side dish for a cold-weather roast. In an Italian home, stuffed mushrooms would typically appear as part of an antipasto spread, and they were always a vehicle for leftovers, combining a bit of pancetta, sausage, or other meat with an extender like bread crumbs. I've cut back on the bread crumbs a bit here and added some sautéed greens and mushrooms to the mix to up the health benefits.

Serves
4 TO 6

16 cremini mushrooms
(about two 8-ounce packages)

4 tablespoons extra-virgin olive oil

1 shallot, minced

1 garlic clove, minced

½ teaspoon kosher salt

½ cup shredded greens, such as
kale, chard, or spinach

¼ cup Garlicky Bread Crumbs
(page 47)

⅓ cup freshly grated pecorino
cheese

Preheat the oven to 400°F.

Wipe the mushrooms clean and remove the stems. Chop 4 of the mushrooms very finely. Arrange the rest in a 9 × 13-inch baking dish and set aside.

In a medium skillet, heat 2 tablespoons of the oil over medium-high heat. Add the shallot and chopped mushrooms and cook, stirring, until the vegetables are very soft, about 6 minutes. Stir in the garlic and salt, then add the greens and stir until they have wilted and most of the liquid has evaporated, 2 or 3 minutes. Stir in the bread crumbs and ¼ cup of the cheese.

Stuff the mushrooms with the filling and sprinkle with the remaining cheese. Drizzle with the remaining 2 tablespoons oil.

Bake until the mushrooms are tender, about 25 minutes. Serve warm.

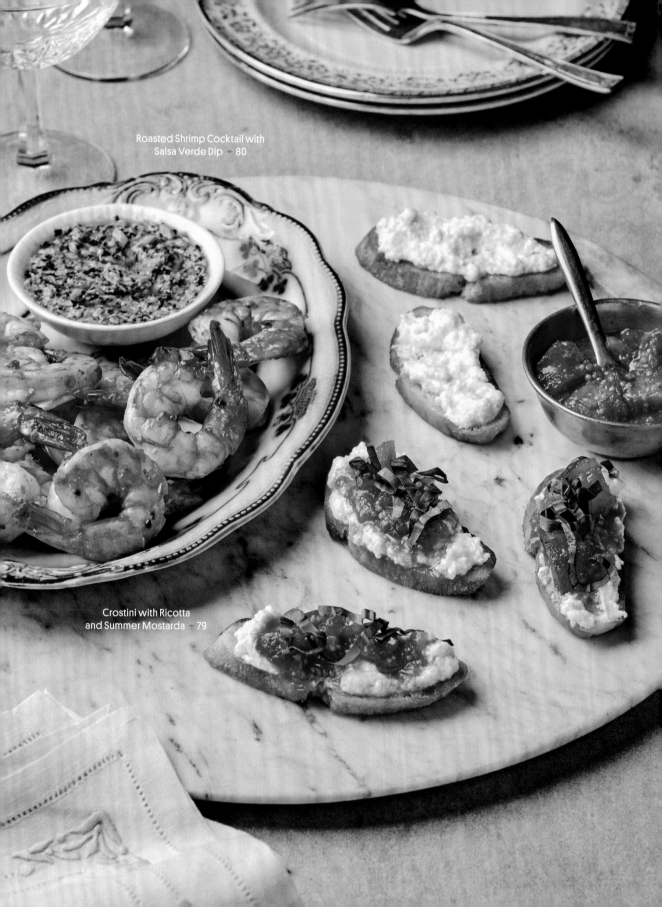

Roasted Shrimp Cocktail with
Salsa Verde Dip ~ 80

Crostini with Ricotta
and Summer Mostarda ~ 79

Crostini WITH **Ricotta**, TWO WAYS

These crostini are one reason I keep a container of ricotta cheese on hand: Souped up with a bit of salt and lemon zest, it makes the perfect base layer for easy and elegant crostini at the drop of a hat. If you have just about any of the condiments in Chapter 1: Flavor Starts Here [page 43] ready to go, you've got yourself a cocktail treat in minutes. The mostarda and peperonata are my favorites, but a drizzle of chile garlic oil, a dollop of olive relish or salsa verde—any of these would be delicious, no-fuss toppers for an impromptu bite. Use a thin ficelle if you can find one; smaller toasts are less likely to spoil your guests' appetites!

Serves

6 TO 8

½ thin baguette, such as a ficelle

3 tablespoons extra-virgin olive oil, plus more for brushing the bread slices

1 cup ricotta cheese, preferably a fresh imported variety

1 teaspoon grated lemon zest

¼ teaspoon kosher salt

1 cup Summer Mostarda [page 58] and/or 1 cup Peperonata [page 59]

Fresh herbs for garnish, such as thinly sliced mint or basil [for the mostarda] or chopped fresh parsley, oregano, or red pepper flakes [for the peperonata]

Preheat the oven to 400°F.

Slice the baguette diagonally into ¼-inch slices. Brush the slices with olive oil, then arrange them on a baking sheet.

Bake until golden brown, 10 to 12 minutes. Set aside to cool.

In a bowl, whisk together the ricotta, lemon zest, the 3 tablespoons oil, and salt. Smear a generous tablespoon of the ricotta on each bread slice, then top with your choice of condiment. Garnish and serve.

Roasted Shrimp Cocktail

WITH SALSA VERDE DIP

If there is one appetizer that never fails to hit, it's shrimp cocktail. I much prefer it when the shrimp are warm, rather than rubbery and cold from the fridge, and this one has all kinds of heat: from the broiler, from the chile garlic oil, and from a bit of horseradish in the dip for good measure.

Serves
6 TO 8

1 pound extra-large shrimp, peeled and deveined

2 tablespoons Calabrian Chile Garlic Oil (page 50)

½ lemon

1 cup Kale Salsa Verde (page 54)

2 tablespoons prepared horseradish

Preheat the broiler with a rack set 6 inches below the heat source.

In a bowl, toss together the shrimp and chile garlic oil to coat. Spread the shrimp on a sheet pan.

Broil without turning until the shrimp are opaque and browned on the edges, about 5 minutes; don't overcook!

Squeeze the lemon over the shrimp and arrange on a serving platter.

In a small bowl, stir the salsa verde and horseradish together and nestle the mixture among the shrimp. Serve warm or at room temperature.

Crunchy Roasted Butter Beans

I got the idea for these crackly tidbits from a side dish I had at Il Buco al Mare, a wonderful Italian restaurant in the Hamptons. Their beans were deep-fried and out of this world, but my sheet pan version is nearly as addictively crisp and couldn't be easier to make. Just a teensy bit of whole wheat flour and my handy-dandy seasoned salt transform a plain-Jane can of beans into a poppable cocktail nibble. These don't store well, so eat 'em up the day you make 'em!

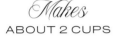

Makes
ABOUT 2 CUPS

1 (15-ounce) can butter beans or cannellini beans, drained

1 tablespoon whole wheat flour

2½ teaspoons GDL Seasoned Salt (page 48)

½ teaspoon garlic powder

2½ tablespoons extra-virgin olive oil

Position a rack in the center of the oven and preheat the oven to 450°F. Line a sheet pan with parchment paper.

Place the beans in a bowl and sprinkle with the flour, 2 teaspoons of the seasoned salt, and the garlic powder. Toss with a fork to distribute. Spread the beans evenly on the prepared pan and drizzle with 1½ tablespoons of the oil. (See Hint.)

Roast until puffed open and crisp, 25 to 30 minutes (a few minutes less for cannellini beans). You don't need to toss or turn them.

Drizzle with the remaining 1 tablespoon oil and sprinkle with the remaining ½ teaspoon seasoned salt. Serve warm.

HINT HINT ◆ An inexpensive squirt bottle is really handy for controlling the amount of oil you are drizzling on your food because the oil comes out in a finer stream than the plastic nozzle on your big bottle allows, which lets you direct it more accurately.

Artichoke Dip

WITH WHITE BEANS

Creamy bean dips are one of my go-to ways for using healthy beans because they taste rich even when made without a lot of fat or dairy. This is an Italian version of a spinach dip, similar to many dips popular in the North of Italy, where they are usually served with crudités. I like my dips on the chunkier side, whether it's guacamole or this cheesy veggie mixture. It is good hot or cold, and the crumbled prosciutto topping is optional, but it adds a nice crunch.

Serves
6 TO 8

- 4 slices prosciutto (optional)

- 1 (12-ounce) package frozen artichoke hearts, thawed

- 1 (15-ounce) can cannellini beans, drained and rinsed

- 1 cup freshly grated pecorino cheese

- ½ cup torn fresh basil leaves

- 1 teaspoon grated lemon zest

- 1 tablespoon fresh lemon juice

- 2 teaspoons kosher salt

- ½ teaspoon freshly ground black pepper

- ¼ cup extra-virgin olive oil, plus more for drizzling

- Toasted country bread, crostini, or vegetable spears, for dipping

Position a rack in the center of the oven and preheat the oven to 375°F. Line a sheet pan with parchment paper.

If using the prosciutto, lay the slices in a single layer on the lined pan and bake until crisp, 10 to 12 minutes. Set aside to cool, leaving the oven on.

In a food processor, combine the artichoke hearts, beans, pecorino, basil, lemon zest and juice, salt, and pepper. Pulse on and off just until the mixture is combined. With the machine running, slowly add the olive oil.

Spoon the dip into an ovenproof crock or small serving bowl and bake until heated through, about 15 minutes.

Crumble the prosciutto and sprinkle on top. Drizzle with oil and serve with your choice of dippers.

Pinzimonio

WITH FANCY CRUDITÉS

In some Italian restaurants, especially in Sicily, you are offered a small bowl of flavored oil with fresh vegetables to enjoy as you peruse the menu. The presentation is simplicity itself, and it is such a light, healthy, and refreshing way to start a meal. Remember this the next time you have unexpected guests; if you don't have beautiful vegetables, serve it with crackers or bread for dipping.

Serves
4 TO 6

½ cup extra-virgin olive oil

2 teaspoons GDL Seasoned Salt (page 48)

Juice of ½ lemon

Assorted raw vegetables, the prettiest you can find: breakfast radishes, Romanesco florets, rainbow carrot spears, endive or Treviso leaves, and so on

In a small bowl, stir together the oil, seasoned salt, and lemon juice, mixing until combined. Place the bowl in the center of a serving platter and surround with the raw vegetables.

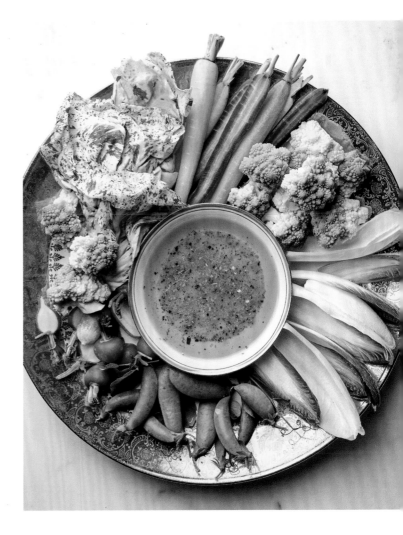

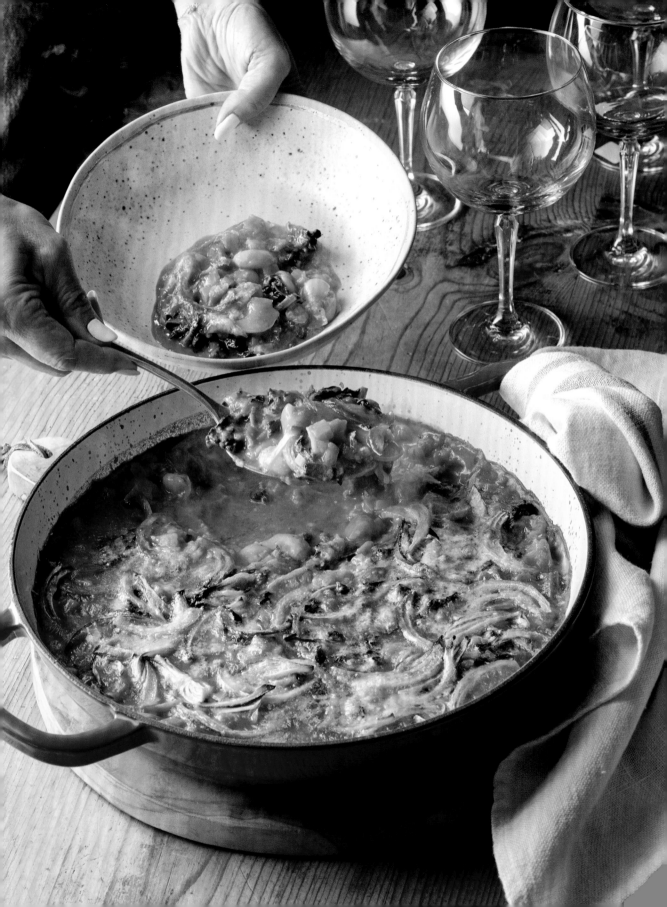

Three

Soups & Main Course Salads

Green Stracciatella 88

Rosemary Lentil Soup
with Porcini 90

Winter Beans AND Greens Soup 91

Green Gazpacho 92

Siena-Style Ribollita 95

Zucchini Artichoke Soup
with Pasta Mista 96

Creamy Kale Caesar
with Shrimp 97

Cauliflower Zuppa
Toscana 99

Baby Gems *with* Avocado
AND PARM DRESSING 100

Grilled Endive Salad
with Citrus AND Pancetta 103

Salmon Panzanella 104

Tuna Salad
with White Beans AND Olives 107

Fregola Salad *with*
OLIVE DRESSING AND CHICKPEAS 108

IT'S NO EXAGGERATION
to say that salads

are one of my basic food groups, followed closely by vegetable-forward soups. These are the dishes that just make me feel good, and they are so wholesome, nutritionally dense, and low in calories that I can eat as much of them as I want without having to think too much about it. With all that going for them, it's no surprise that these are recipes I come back to again and again.

I like to eat some raw vegetables every day, and nine times out of ten that means a salad. In Italy, salads are usually found on the antipasto table, but living in California and having so much great fresh produce available all year long has normalized the concept of salad as a main course for me. Fortunately, few things make me happier (or hungrier) than sitting down to a gorgeous plate of vegetables or grains, fortified with a bit of cheese, beans, or meat for protein, all brought together with a really punchy dressing.

Of course, nothing partners better with a salad than a bowl of nourishing, warming soup. Soups are a really big part of the Italian diet, especially in the North, where temperatures can dip quite a bit lower than they do in the Southern regions, and hearty soups are essential comfort food. I got my love of soup from my aunt Raffy, who is famous in our family for cooking up huge pots every Sunday, which she then portions out and freezes for future meals. (If you look in her freezer, it's like a soup-themed pop-up shop!) I always resolve to do this myself, but I'm generally not disciplined enough to plan my week that well; plus, when soups are as delicious as these, they tend to disappear before I can get them in the freezer.

Both salads and soups are very amenable to leftovers, and many, like the classic ribollita or panzanella salads, were invented as a way to repurpose stale hunks of bread, a handful of beans or greens, even cooked pasta. While I like to use chicken broth as a base for my soups to give them more depth and body, you'll see that meat (often something from the pork family) is used almost as a seasoning rather than a main ingredient in all the recipes in this chapter. For that reason, centering one meal of the day around a bowl of soup or a lovely big salad is a smart, convenient way to eat if you are trying to limit the amount of meat in your diet.

Green Stracciatella

Not every recipe is meant to be the centerpiece of a menu for entertaining. This is something to make when you are feeling a little run-down. Pantry ingredients are the heroes of this quickly assembled soup: eggs, grated cheese, and well-flavored chicken broth. A few handfuls of baby spinach give it a lovely color and, of course, additional nutrients. Some recipes call for wilting the spinach right into the broth, but I have never really loved the texture; instead, I puree the spinach and combine it with the eggs to create puffy green curds of cheesy eggs. Adding shredded chicken isn't really traditional, but it makes this comforting soup even more satisfying. I've written this recipe to serve two, as it's the perfect impromptu lunch or late-night snack.

Serves

2

◆

2 cups (lightly packed) baby spinach

4 cups Parmesan Chicken Broth (page 64) or low-sodium store-bought chicken broth (see Hint)

2 large eggs

½ cup freshly grated Parmigiano-Reggiano cheese, plus more for serving

¼ teaspoon kosher salt

1½ cups shredded chicken breast (optional)

2 small lemon wedges

In a blender, combine the spinach with ¼ cup of the chicken broth. Puree until the spinach is very smooth and bright green. Transfer to a medium bowl, then add the eggs, Parmigiano, and salt and stir gently with a fork until the eggs are broken up and the color is uniform; don't beat too vigorously, as you don't want to incorporate a lot of air into the eggs.

In a saucepan, bring the remaining 3¾ cups chicken broth to a gentle simmer over medium heat. Give the broth a good stir, creating an eddy in the center of the pot, and gently stream in the egg mixture. Let it cook without stirring for about 2 minutes, until the eggs have set. Add the shredded chicken (if using) and simmer until heated through, 2 or 3 minutes.

Ladle into serving bowls, breaking up the eggs into clumps. Serve with a squeeze of lemon juice and a sprinkle of additional Parmigiano.

HINT HINT ◆ If you are using store-bought broth, boost its flavor by simmering it with a piece of Parmigiano rind, a sprig of fresh thyme or parsley, ½ teaspoon salt, and a garlic clove for 15 to 20 minutes, then proceed with the recipe as above.

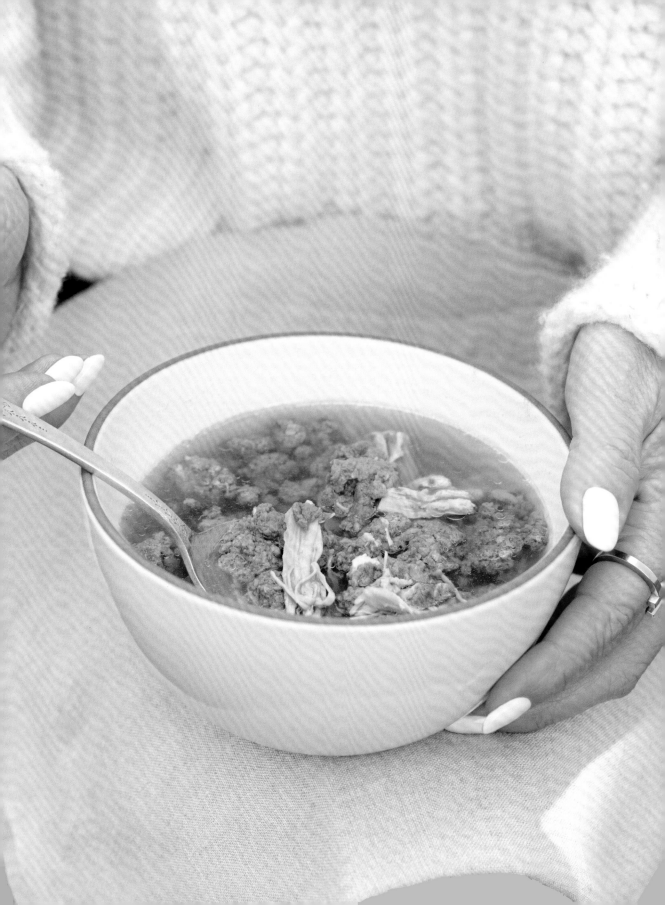

Rosemary Lentil Soup
WITH Porcini

Lentil soup can be . . . just fine, or it can be great, full of interesting textures and flavors, like this one. The earthy flavors of rosemary, lentils, and dried mushrooms combine to make a soup that is incredibly hearty and satisfying even though it is completely vegan. Lemon and the bitter edge of broccoli rabe add a note of brightness. I find it plenty satisfying as is, but it would also be delicious with bits of sausage or kielbasa stirred in, or a sprinkle of grated pecorino if you aren't eating strictly plant-based.

Serves
6

1 bunch broccoli rabe, stems trimmed

2 tablespoons extra-virgin olive oil, plus more for drizzling

1 cup chopped onions

½ cup chopped celery

1 cup chopped carrots

1 garlic clove, chopped

1 teaspoon kosher salt

¼ teaspoon red pepper flakes

2 tablespoons tomato paste

1 tablespoon plus 1 teaspoon chopped fresh rosemary, plus more for serving

1½ cups lentils

1 ounce dried porcini mushrooms, crumbled

1 lemon, halved

In a heavy soup pot, bring 4 cups well-salted water to a boil over high heat. Add the broccoli rabe and blanch for 3 minutes. Drain the broccoli rabe, refresh under cold water, and set aside in a colander while you make the soup.

Add the oil to the same pot and place over medium heat. Add the onions, celery, carrots, and garlic. Season with ½ teaspoon of the salt and the pepper flakes and cook, stirring frequently, until softened, about 6 minutes. Stir in the tomato paste and rosemary and cook until the tomato paste has darkened to a rich red, about another minute.

Stir in the lentils, dried mushrooms, the remaining ½ teaspoon salt, and 6 cups water. Bring the soup to a boil. Add the lemon halves, reduce the heat to low, cover, and simmer until the lentils are quite tender, about 25 minutes.

Cut the broccoli rabe into 1-inch pieces, add to the soup, and heat through. Squeeze the lemon halves into the soup and discard the rinds.

Serve drizzled with a bit more olive oil and a pinch of chopped rosemary.

Winter Beans AND Greens Soup

Similar to my Siena-Style Ribollita [page 95] but a lot quicker to make, this hits all the H's: hearty, healthy, and homey. I like to make it when I've cooked up a batch of dried beans [see Hint] because the cooking liquid adds body and richness, but canned cannellini beans are a perfectly acceptable shortcut. Either way, it will be ready to serve in about 30 minutes. This is the kind of soup my aunt Raffy often makes on a Sunday afternoon to eat throughout the week, because it provides a simple, nutritious meal served with a salad at the end of a long workday.

Serves

4

❧

2 tablespoons extra-virgin olive oil, plus more for drizzling

1 onion, chopped

1 celery stalk, chopped

1 carrot, peeled and chopped

2 garlic cloves, smashed and peeled

1½ teaspoons kosher salt

½ teaspoon red pepper flakes [optional]

3 cups cooked cannellini beans with a little of their cooking liquid [see Hint]

4 cups Parmesan Chicken Broth [page 64] or low-sodium store-bought chicken broth

1 head escarole or 1 [5-ounce] package [about 6 cups] baby spinach, chopped

Freshly grated pecorino cheese, for serving

In a medium Dutch oven, heat the oil over medium-high heat. Add the onion, celery, carrot, and garlic. Season with the salt and cook, stirring often, until the vegetables are starting to soften, about 4 minutes. Add the pepper flakes (if using) and cannellini beans and liquid and stir to combine.

Add the broth and bring to a simmer. Reduce the heat to medium and simmer gently for 5 minutes. Stir in the escarole and continue to cook until the escarole is tender, about 5 minutes (if using spinach, you will only need to cook it for a minute or two).

Serve topped with a drizzle of oil and a generous sprinkle of pecorino.

HINT HINT ◆ Cooking dried beans is an imprecise art; depending on their age and size they can take as little as 50 minutes to cook and as long as 2 hours. For a large batch to use in multiple recipes, combine 4 cups dried beans such as cannellini with 4 garlic cloves, 2 tablespoons extra-virgin olive oil, 2 bay leaves, and 12 cups water in a large pot. Bring to a boil over medium-high heat, then reduce the heat and cook at a gentle simmer, partially covered, until tender. Start checking the beans after about 1 hour; they should be just tender all the way through but not falling apart. If they are still hard or chalky tasting, keep cooking, testing every 15 minutes or so. When they are ready, stir in 1½ teaspoons kosher salt. Cool to room temperature before refrigerating for up to 5 days.

Green Gazpacho

If you associate gazpacho primarily with Spanish cuisine, you're not wrong—it's practically the national dish. But Italians have been drawing on Spain's tradition of chilled vegetable soups for centuries and it's my preferred way to eat soup in the summer. My version is bright green, which makes it as refreshing visually as it is on the palate. Green grapes and a tiny bit of chile paste make it extra vibrant, with a lovely balance of sweet, sharp, and spicy flavors.

Serves
4

2 pints yellow tomatoes,
such as Sungold

2 heaping cups chopped cucumber
(from 3 Persian/mini cucumbers
or 1 hothouse cucumber)

1 small or ½ large sweet onion,
chopped

2 cups (loosely packed)
baby spinach

½ cup fresh basil leaves,
plus more for serving

1 cup green grapes

½ teaspoon Calabrian chile paste
(optional)

1¾ teaspoons kosher salt,
plus more to taste

3 heaping cups cubed ciabatta
(about 3 thick slices)

1½ tablespoons extra-virgin
olive oil, plus more for serving

½ teaspoon dried Sicilian oregano

Balsamic vinegar, for serving

In a blender, combine the tomatoes, cucumber, onion, spinach, basil, grapes, chile paste, and 1¼ teaspoons of the salt and blend until nearly smooth. Taste and add a bit more salt if needed. Refrigerate for at least 2 hours and up to 3 days.

Preheat the oven to 400°F.

Place the bread cubes on a sheet pan. Drizzle with the oil and sprinkle with the oregano and the remaining ½ teaspoon salt. Toss with your hands to coat. Bake the bread cubes until golden brown, about 15 minutes, tossing once.

To serve, ladle the chilled soup into bowls and drizzle each serving with a bit of olive oil and balsamic vinegar. Top with a few croutons and some basil.

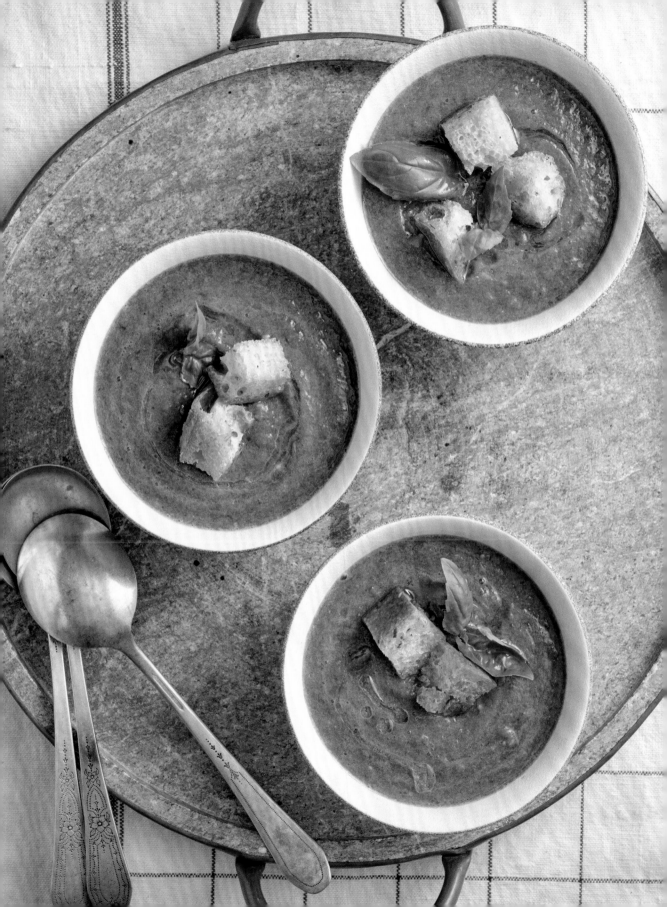

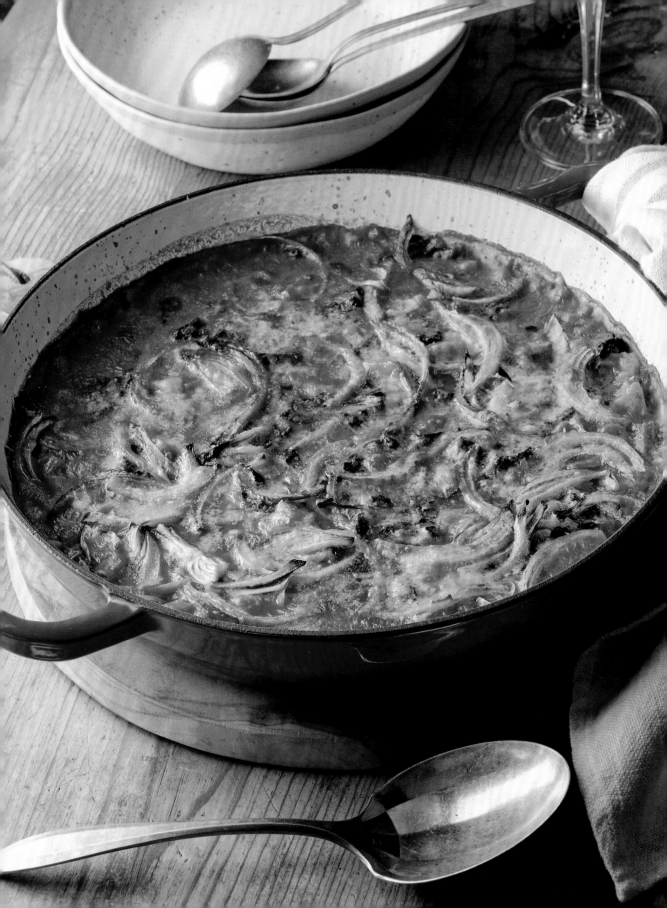

Siena-Style Ribollita

Soup doesn't get more comforting—or filling—than this. A rich mixture of beans and vegetables slow-cooked with a chunk of Parmesan until soft, the soup takes on the texture of a porridge when bits of stale bread are simmered into the broth. In Siena it is served with a delectable caramelized onion and cheese crust that is reminiscent of French onion soup, and that's my favorite way to serve it. This makes a generous quantity and takes a little more effort than some recipes in this book, so I like to bust it out for a casual gathering, like game night or my Oscars viewing party.

Serves
4 TO 6

◆

4 tablespoons extra-virgin olive oil, plus more for serving

1 cup chopped yellow onions

½ cup chopped fennel or celery

½ cup chopped carrots

2 garlic cloves, chopped

Kosher salt and freshly ground black pepper

1 (15-ounce) can cannellini or butter beans, undrained

1 large bunch lacinato (Tuscan) kale, tough ends trimmed, chopped into bite-size pieces

2 cups low-sodium beef broth

½ cup passata (tomato puree)

2-ounce chunk Parmigiano-Reggiano cheese, broken into pieces

2 ciabatta rolls, preferably a day or two old, cubed (about 2 cups)

1 tablespoon red wine vinegar

1 small red onion, very thinly sliced

⅓ cup freshly grated Parmigiano-Reggiano cheese

Fennel fronds, for garnish

In a Dutch oven, heat 2 tablespoons of the oil over medium-low heat. Add the yellow onions, fennel, carrots, garlic, and salt and pepper to taste. Sauté until softened, about 6 minutes. Add half the beans to the pot and use a potato masher to crush them into a rough puree. Add the remaining beans and their liquid, the kale, broth, passata, Parmigiano pieces, and 2 cups water. Bring to a boil. Reduce the heat to low, cover, and simmer for 15 minutes.

Preheat the oven to 450°F.

Stir the bread cubes into the Dutch oven, making sure they are submerged in liquid, then cover and simmer until the kale is very soft and the bread is falling apart, another 15 minutes.

Stir the soup briskly with a whisk to break up the bread cubes and cheese and to create a thick, porridge-like texture. Stir in the vinegar and more salt and pepper to taste.

Arrange the red onion slices over the soup in a single layer and sprinkle evenly with the grated Parmigiano. Drizzle with the remaining 2 tablespoons olive oil.

Transfer to the oven and bake, uncovered, until the onion and cheese are golden brown, about 20 minutes.

Serve topped with fennel fronds and another drizzle of oil, making sure that each serving gets some of the crusty topping.

Zucchini Artichoke Soup
WITH Pasta Mista

Zucchini doesn't end up in the soup pot very often in this country, but Italians know it cooks down to a lovely pale green with a smooth, almost creamy texture. *Pasta mista* means "mixed pasta," a hodgepodge of mismatched shapes and sizes that mimics the assorted odds and ends of pasta most Italians have kicking around their pantries and that commonly get thrown in for a bit of bulk. I like to cook the pasta separately and then let it cook briefly in the soup. However, if I know I won't be serving it all when it's freshly made, I'll add the pasta to each portion as I serve, because the leftovers will continue to absorb liquid and become too soft. You can also cook the pasta right in the soup, simmering it for about 5 minutes or until tender. Be sure to choose slender, young zucchini for this, as they will have the fewest seeds.

Serves
6 TO 8

◆

¼ cup extra-virgin olive oil, plus more for drizzling

2 leeks, white and pale green parts only, chopped

2 garlic cloves, minced

6 slender zucchini, thinly sliced

2 (13-ounce) jars water-packed quartered artichoke hearts, drained

Kosher salt and freshly ground black pepper

10 cups Savory Vegetable Broth (page 65) or low-sodium store-bought vegetable broth

1 tablespoon chopped fresh thyme leaves

4 ounces mixed short pasta shapes

Freshly grated Parmigiano-Reggiano cheese, for serving

In a large heavy pot, heat the oil over medium heat. Add the leeks and sauté until translucent, about 8 minutes. Add the garlic and sauté until tender, about 2 minutes. Stir in the zucchini and artichokes. Season the vegetables with salt and pepper. Sauté until the zucchini is tender, about 10 minutes.

Add the vegetable broth and thyme, cover the pot, and bring to a simmer over medium heat. Reduce the heat to medium-low and simmer gently until the flavors develop, stirring occasionally, about 20 minutes.

Meanwhile, bring a large pot of salted water to a boil. Add the pasta and cook until al dente. Drain the pasta and stir into the soup, simmering together for a minute or two to marry the flavors.

Ladle the soup into bowls. Sprinkle with Parmigiano, drizzle with a bit of oil, and serve.

Creamy Kale Caesar
WITH **Shrimp**

This is the kind of kitchen math I love: 1 dark leafy green + (condiments × 2) = 1 Super-Italian salad in minutes! It's creamy and crunchy and full of big, big flavors. I find it equally satisfying on its own or topped with a simple grilled chicken breast, a salmon fillet, or shrimp, as here. Don't punt on the step of massaging the greens, especially if you are using kale; it really makes it much more tender.

Serves
4 TO 6

1 bunch lacinato (Tuscan) kale, stripped off the center ribs and chopped, or 1 (5-ounce) package baby kale (about 6 cups)

2 tablespoons extra-virgin olive oil

1 tablespoon fresh lemon juice

¾ teaspoon kosher salt

1 pound large shrimp, peeled and deveined

½ teaspoon GDL Seasoned Salt (page 48)

¼ cup Caesar Aioli (page 53)

½ cup Garlicky Bread Crumbs (page 47), plus more for serving

Shaved Parmigiano-Reggiano cheese, for serving

Preheat the broiler.

Place the kale in a large bowl and drizzle with 1 tablespoon of the oil and the lemon juice. Sprinkle with the kosher salt. Using your hand or something blunt like the end of a wooden rolling pin, squeeze or bruise the greens to tenderize them.

Toss the shrimp with the seasoned salt and the remaining 1 tablespoon oil and spread on a sheet pan. Broil the shrimp without turning until there are a few golden spots on the edges and they are cooked through, about 3 minutes.

Add the aioli to the kale and use tongs to toss and mix, coating the leaves evenly. Sprinkle with the bread crumbs and mix again.

Mound the salad on serving plates, topping each portion with another sprinkle of bread crumbs and some shaved Parmigiano. Arrange the warm shrimp on the salads and serve.

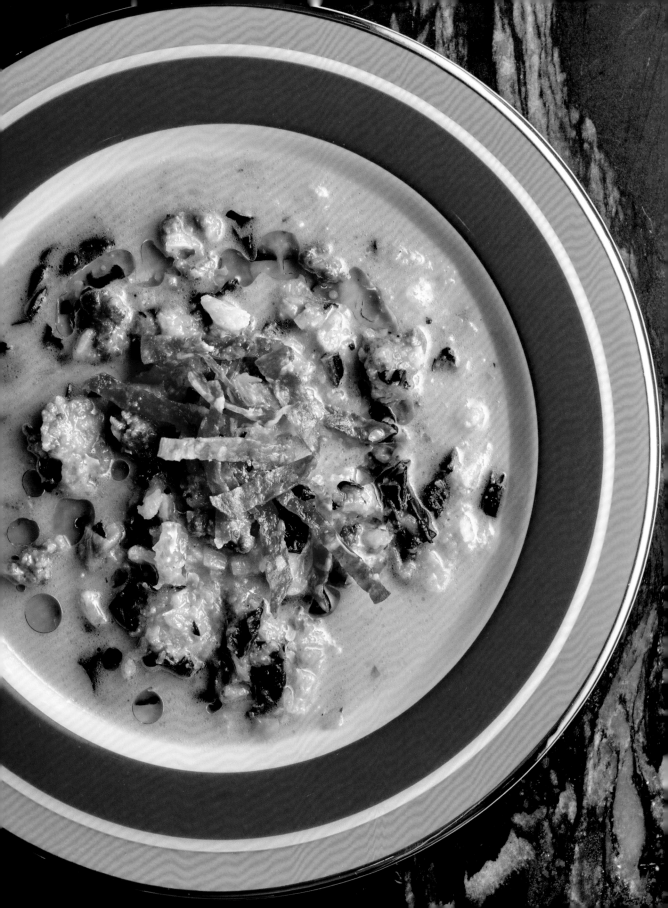

Cauliflower Zuppa Toscana

You would swear there is dairy in this rich, creamy soup, but other than a bit of Parm rind in the broth, it is completely dairy-free. Nonetheless it's one of the most warming, soothing cold-weather soups I can think of. The garnish is, of course, optional, but it adds a nice textural and visual contrast.

Serves

4

1 tablespoon extra-virgin olive oil, plus more for drizzling

8 ounces sweet Italian turkey or pork sausage (about 2 links), casings removed

1 small leek, white part only, halved lengthwise and sliced ¼ inch thick

1 large Yukon Gold potato, cut into ½-inch cubes

½ head cauliflower (about ½ pound), chopped into small pieces

1 teaspoon kosher salt, plus more to taste

1 bay leaf

4 cups Parmesan Chicken Broth (page 64) or low-sodium store-bought chicken broth plus a 2-inch piece Parmigiano-Reggiano rind

2 cups chopped curly or lacinato (Tuscan) kale (2 ounces)

2 slices salami or prosciutto (optional), cut into thin strips

In a heavy-bottomed saucepan or small soup pot, heat the oil over medium heat. Add the sausage to the pan, breaking the meat into bite-size bits with a wooden spoon. Cook, stirring often, until the sausage is no longer pink, 4 to 5 minutes. Remove the sausage to a plate and add the leek to the pan, cooking and stirring until softened, 3 to 4 minutes.

Add the potato, cauliflower, salt, bay leaf, and broth to the pan (plus the Parm rind if using store-bought broth) and bring to a boil. Cook until the potatoes are nearly tender and the cauliflower is falling apart, about 10 minutes.

Use an immersion blender or potato masher to puree some of the vegetables into the broth until thick and creamy. Add the sausage and kale and cook over low heat until the kale is wilted and the sausage is heated through, about 4 minutes. Add a bit more salt to taste if needed.

If garnishing with the salami, warm it in a small skillet over medium heat until the fat has rendered and the strips are crispy, just a minute or two.

Ladle the soup into bowls, top with the crispy salami (if using) and a drizzle of olive oil, and serve hot.

Baby Gems WITH Avocado

I had to include at least one nod to my California lifestyle, and this green-on-green-on-green salad fits the bill perfectly. This would make a pretty dish for a ladies' luncheon with the addition of grilled salmon or poached shrimp.

Serves

4

8 slices prosciutto

4 heads Baby Gem lettuce, quartered lengthwise

2 avocados, each cut into 8 wedges

2 radishes, thinly sliced

1 cup Do-It-All Parmesan Dressing [page 51]

Position a rack in the upper third of the oven and preheat the oven to 400°F. Line a sheet pan with parchment paper.

Arrange the prosciutto on the lined pan in a single layer. Bake until crisp, 8 to 10 minutes. Let the prosciutto cool on the pan.

Arrange 4 lettuce quarters on each of four serving plates and tuck the avocado wedges among them. Sprinkle on the radishes.

Drizzle the salads with the dressing, then shred a couple of prosciutto slices over each serving.

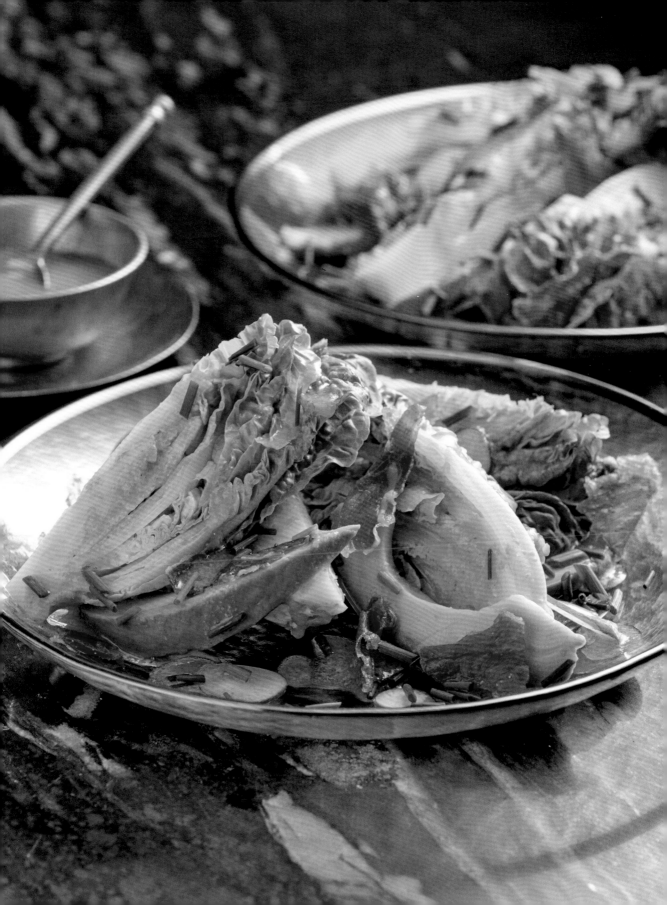

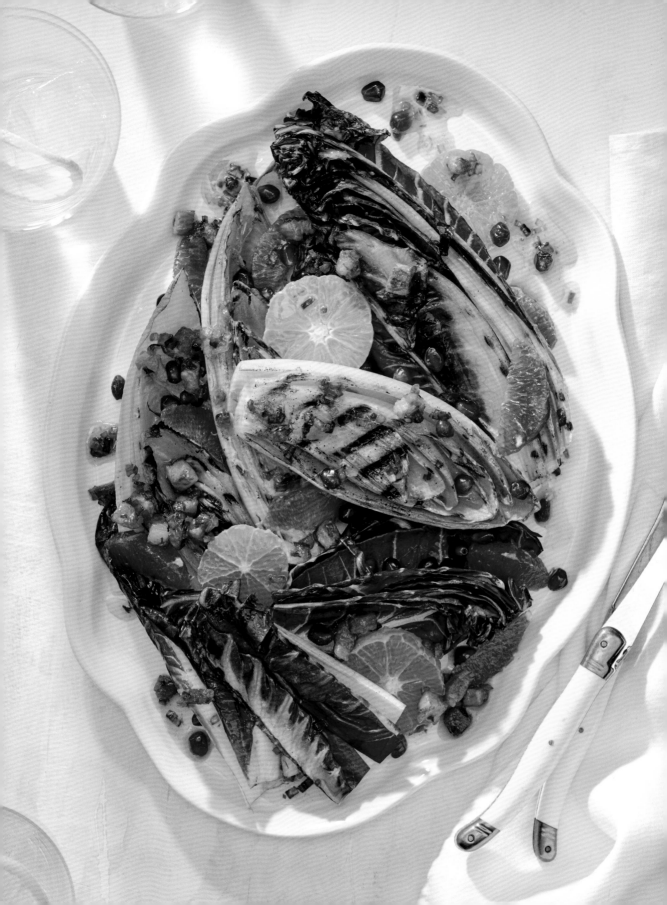

Grilled Endive Salad
WITH **Citrus** AND **Pancetta**

Winter is when citrus fruits are at their best and most varied, and it's also the right season for bitter greens, also called chicories. Together they make a perfect pair, especially when the greens get a kiss from a grill pan to soften them and bring out their sweetness. A bit of salty pancetta, though not essential if you want to keep things vegetarian, does add a nice crunch and chew that I really enjoy. I serve this as a lunch dish, but in smaller portions it would also be a wonderful complement to a rich or heavy meal, as the bright, somewhat astringent flavors cut through the fattiness of roasted or stewed meats.

Serves

4

❖

FOR THE GRILLED CHICORIES

3 red or white endives, halved lengthwise

1 large head Treviso, quartered lengthwise

2 tablespoons extra-virgin olive oil

½ teaspoon kosher salt

FOR THE DRESSING

¼ pound pancetta, cut into ⅓-inch dice

3 tablespoons extra-virgin olive oil

1 shallot, chopped

1 teaspoon Dijon mustard

1 tablespoon white wine vinegar

FOR ASSEMBLY

1 blood or Cara Cara orange, separated into segments

1 clementine, peeled and sliced in rounds

2 tablespoons pomegranate seeds

Grill the chicories: Preheat a grill or ridged grill pan over medium-high heat.

Drizzle the endives and Treviso with the oil and season with the salt. Place the chicories on the grill and cook until lightly marked with grill lines, about 2 minutes. Turn the pieces and grill for another 2 minutes. Use tongs to transfer the pieces to a serving platter.

While the chicories grill, make the dressing: In a small skillet, place the pancetta and 1 tablespoon of the oil over medium heat. Cook, stirring often, until the fat is rendered and the pancetta is starting to crisp around the edges, about 5 minutes. Add the shallot and cook until the shallot is soft and the pancetta is fully crisp, about 3 minutes longer. Remove from the heat and cool slightly. Stir in the remaining 2 tablespoons oil, the mustard, and the vinegar.

To assemble: Scatter the citrus over the grilled chicories and sprinkle with the pomegranate seeds. Spoon the dressing over the salad and serve warm.

Salmon Panzanella

Italian cooks hate to waste anything, even stale bread, and that economical attitude is the genesis of panzanella salad, a mixture of bread cubes and vegetables tossed with a tangy dressing. They can be made with anything from calamari to corn bread; the only constant is the delicious cubes of toasted bread, which soak up the lemony dressing like little sponges and explode in your mouth with every bite. In Italy, a panzanella would usually be served as a side salad or part of an antipasto spread; I've made it a one-dish meal by adding cooked salmon, and if you have any leftover cooked veggies, by all means, add them, too!

Serves
4 TO 6

1 pound skinless salmon fillet

1 teaspoon GDL Seasoned Salt (page 48)

2 lemons, halved

4 cups 1-inch cubes stale bread

¼ cup plus ⅓ cup extra-virgin olive oil

½ cup freshly grated Parmigiano-Reggiano cheese

1 teaspoon kosher salt

2 cups cherry tomatoes, halved

½ cup pitted Castelvetrano olives, halved

3 cups baby arugula

½ cup fresh basil leaves

Preheat the broiler with a rack about 6 inches below the heat source.

Pat the salmon dry and sprinkle with the seasoned salt. Place the fish on a sheet pan skin side down. Broil the fish without turning until the top has a nice golden crust and the salmon is cooked through, 10 to 12 minutes, depending on the thickness. Squeeze the juice of ½ lemon over the salmon and set aside to cool while you prepare the salad.

Reduce the oven temperature to 400°F. Line a sheet pan with parchment paper.

In a large bowl, combine the bread cubes, ¼ cup of the oil, the Parmigiano, and ½ teaspoon of the kosher salt and toss to coat. Scatter the cubes on the lined pan and bake until golden brown and crispy, about 12 minutes.

Return the toasted cubes to the bowl and add the tomatoes, olives, and arugula. Tear the basil into small pieces and add it to the bowl.

Juice the remaining lemons into a small bowl and season with the remaining ½ teaspoon kosher salt. Whisk in the remaining ⅓ cup oil. Drizzle the dressing over the salad and toss to combine. Use two forks to break the salmon into bite-size pieces and add to the bowl. Toss once more and serve.

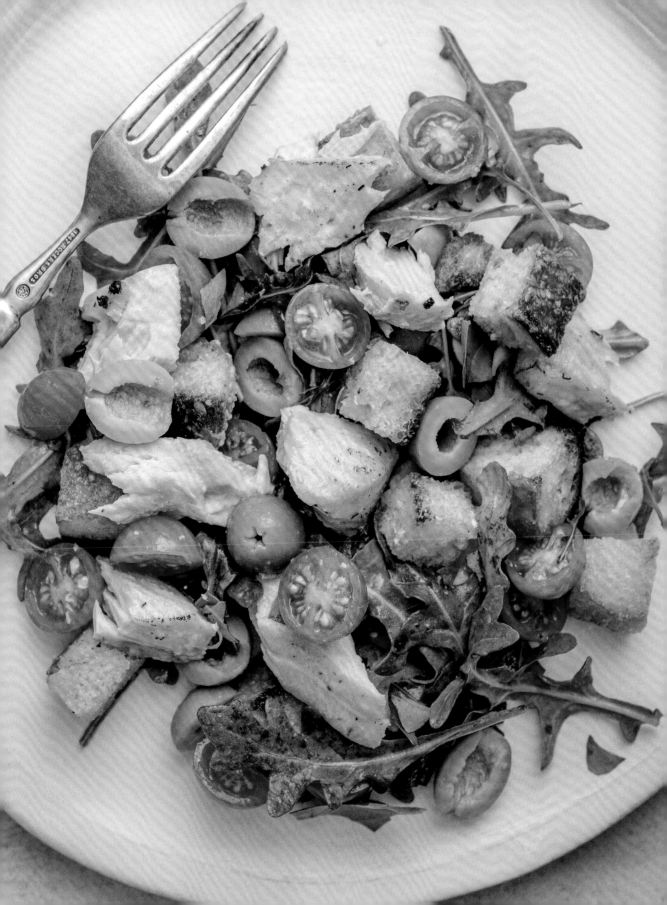

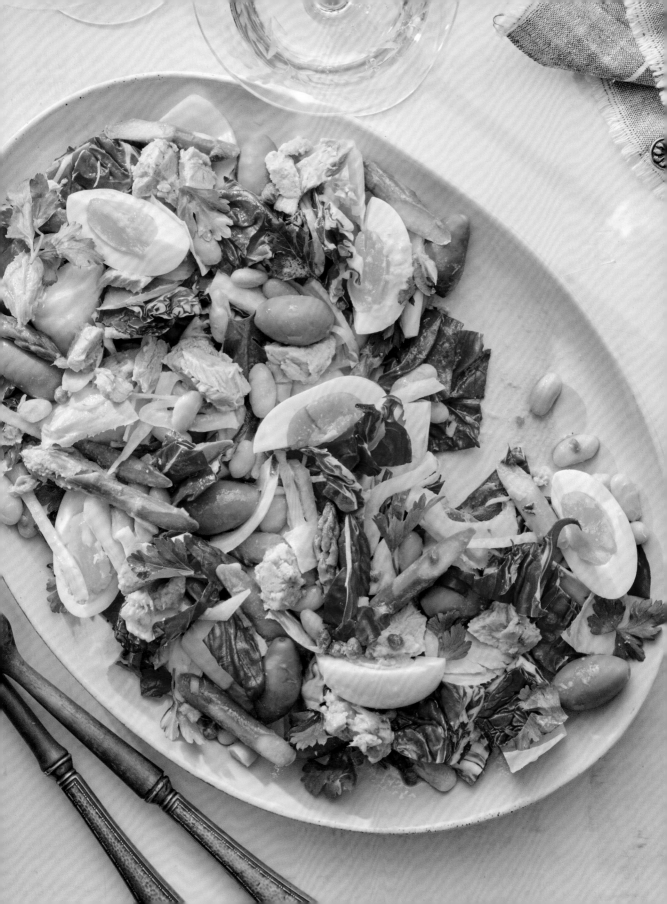

Tuna Salad
with **White Beans** and **Olives**

If you asked a Southern Italian cook to whip up a salade Niçoise, the result would probably look a little something like this, a blend of flavorful ingredients with more than enough protein to keep you going for hours. It's sturdy enough to pack for a picnic or work lunch, but when I serve it at home, I add a bed of tender arugula to get in even more greens. If you can, opt for imported Italian tuna packed in olive oil, which is so much more flavorful than the water-packed kind. Whole olives on the pit would be most authentic in a salad like this, but if you go that route, be sure to give your guests a heads-up!

Serves

4

◆

1 tablespoon drained capers, chopped

¼ cup fresh lemon juice

2 teaspoons Dijon mustard

½ cup extra-virgin olive oil

1 teaspoon kosher salt, plus more to taste

1 (15-ounce) can cannellini beans, drained and rinsed

2 (5-ounce) cans or 2 (6-ounce) jars tuna packed in olive oil, drained

½ cup Cerignola olives, pitted or whole

2 Belgian endives, cut into 2-inch pieces

1 small head radicchio, cut into 2-inch pieces

1 small fennel bulb (stalks removed), halved and thinly sliced

½ cup (lightly packed) fresh flat-leaf Italian parsley leaves

2 hard-boiled eggs, peeled and quartered

In a large bowl, whisk together the capers, lemon juice, and mustard. Whisk in the oil in a steady stream until emulsified. Whisk in the salt.

Add the beans, tuna, and olives to the dressing, breaking the tuna into bite-size pieces. Toss gently to coat the ingredients with the dressing and set aside to marinate for 15 minutes, or up to 24 hours in the refrigerator.

When ready to serve, arrange the endives, radicchio, and fennel on a platter. Stir the parsley leaves into the tuna mixture and spoon onto the greens. Arrange the eggs atop the salad and serve, sprinkled with salt to taste.

Fregola Salad

WITH OLIVE DRESSING AND CHICKPEAS

We've come a long way since "pasta salad" meant elbow macaroni drowning in mayo, but even so, most pasta salads are more pasta than salad and more often than not, too soggy and bland for my taste. I like to make mine with a small pasta shape, like orzo or, as here, fregola, a small Sardinian pasta similar to an Israeli couscous (a good substitute if you can't find fregola). This is a fairly straightforward salad, with some chickpeas for protein, but you could add cucumber, cooked broccoli, bits of cheese, or tuna to make it even more substantial.

Serves
4 TO 6

1½ cups (about 8 ounces) fregola or Israeli couscous

1 teaspoon kosher salt, plus more to taste

¾ cup Green Olive Relish (page 55)

1 (15-ounce) can chickpeas, drained and rinsed

1½ cups red and yellow grape or cherry tomatoes, halved

2 cups baby arugula

¼ cup extra-virgin olive oil

2 tablespoons red wine vinegar

Freshly ground black pepper

In a saucepan, combine the fregola, salt, and 4 cups water and bring to a boil. Reduce the heat to low, partially cover, and cook until the fregola is tender, about 15 minutes. Drain well, then transfer to a large bowl. Stir in ½ cup of the olive relish until well combined and set aside to cool for at least 15 minutes.

In a medium bowl, combine the chickpeas, tomatoes, arugula, oil, vinegar, and the remaining ¼ cup olive relish.

Add the chickpea mixture to the fregola and combine. Season to taste with salt and pepper and serve at room temperature.

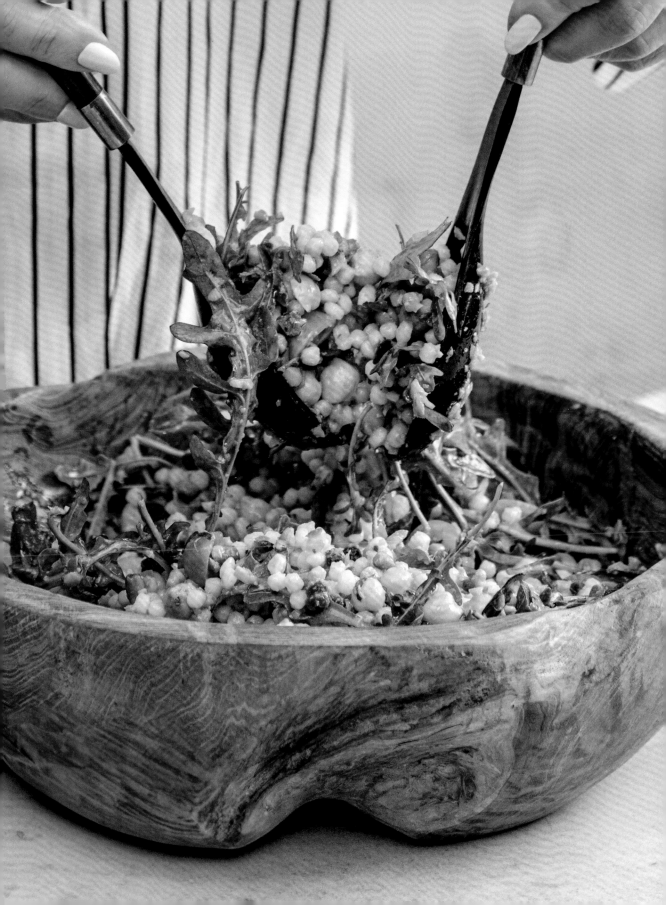

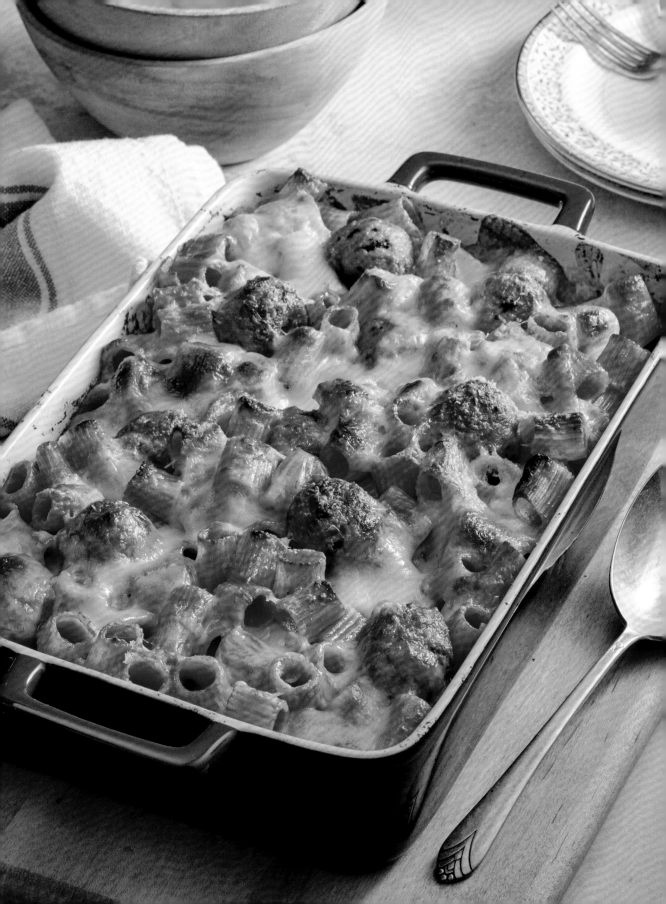

Pasta!

When I sit down to write
A COOKBOOK,

I always put the most thought and time into the pasta chapter because, simply put, pasta is the hallmark of the Italian table. It's also an economical way to serve a lot of people. For my family, there was some form of pasta on the table at nearly every meal and to this day I eat pasta at least three or four times a week. As for so many Italians, it's my starch of choice and I never get tired of dreaming up ways to pair different shapes and sauces with my favorite veggies and proteins. For me, a well-prepared plate of pasta is the very essence of La Dolce Vita: It just makes me happy.

In spending time in different regions of Italy as I sourced ingredients for my website, though, I realized how narrow our impression of pasta is in this country. Like everything else in Italy, pasta preferences are regional. In Rome, many of the pasta sauces are flavored with pork, like pancetta or guanciale; in the South and coastal towns cooks use anchovies to add that deep umami base. And tomato sauce, which Americans associate with spaghetti the way peanut butter goes with jelly, is mostly only paired with pasta in the South; Northerners like their pasta with creamy sauces, often baked with béchamel, and are more likely to include meat in their pasta sauces than those from other areas. Exploring all these regional differences has introduced me to a whole new world of delicious pastas.

Using a variety of shapes and sizes is another aspect of cooking pasta that doesn't always get its due. Each one creates a different chew and gives your dishes more interest, whether it's orecchiette made from the stickier wheat grown in Puglia, or a toothsome spaghetti chitarra from Abruzzo. When I set about developing my own line of pasta, I wanted to include some shapes that I grew up with that are really tough to source in this country. As kids, we were allowed to go to the pantry and pick the shape we wanted to eat that day, and that was part of the excitement of the meal for us. We always chose manfredi lunghi, a long, flat pasta with ruffled edges, like lasagna. I have such sweet memories of watching my grandfather break up the oversized strands to fit into the pot, a ritual I re-enact with Jade today.

Of course, the question that comes up all the time is how I—or anyone—can eat pasta more than occasionally without paying the price of weight gain. I know I've said it a million times, but it all comes down to the quality of the ingredients you use and, perhaps most important, the portion size. A giant bowl of mass-produced pasta drowned in store-bought sauce may be a fast and easy way to fill your belly, but it isn't going to do you any favors nutritionally. In Italian homes, pasta is not traditionally the main course; it's considered the primo, or starter. (When we think of antipasti in the United States we think of cheese boards and charcuterie; in Italy it's usually a small portion of pasta.) I don't prepare multiple courses unless it's a holiday or a special occasion, but rarely do I serve up a huge bowl of pasta on its own for dinner. If I'm serving a simple pasta, I always pair it with some sides—definitely a green—and even a quick protein, like grilled chicken or shrimp. If I don't have a lot of time to think about multiple courses, I pick a pasta dish that includes some protein, for more of a one-pot meal, or I mix and match with some leftover salmon or chicken from the night before. I think it's always better to augment the dish with other ingredients rather than double up on the size of the portions. That way I am covering my nutritional bases without going overboard on carbs.

And regarding portion sizes, we all need to recalibrate our expectations. In many cookbooks 1 pound of pasta is intended to serve 4, which is a *big* portion—much bigger than most Italians consider reasonable, and a lot for the gut to break down. The recipes in this chapter use 1 pound of pasta to serve 6 and depending upon what else is on the table you could even stretch it to serve 8 (or make a half recipe of pasta to serve 4). It may seem skimpy at first if you are accustomed to serving a large plate heaped with pasta, but trust me, 2 ounces is more than enough to satisfy most appetites when accompanied by a side and a salad. To help transition to these more moderate portions, do as I do and scale down your plates to a dessert or salad plate. When you use a big plate, the tendency is to want to fill it up! Before long you'll be wondering how you could ever have consumed the mountain of pasta that once seemed par for the course and loving every bite all the more.

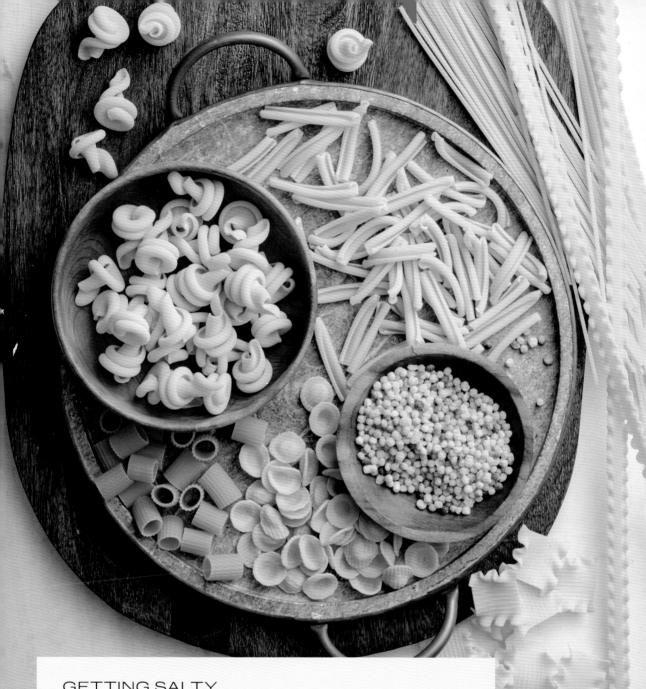

GETTING SALTY

You'll notice that all my pasta recipes direct you to generously salt the water you cook the pasta in, and I cannot stress how important this is. Italians often add a ladle or two of the starchy cooking water to their sauce to make it creamier and help it cling to the pasta. If you don't season the water aggressively—¼ cup of kosher salt is not too much for a pot that holds 8 to 12 quarts of water—not only will your pasta taste bland, but your entire dish will be underseasoned if you are making the sauce with water that's not salty enough. Long story short: Don't be timid when seasoning your pasta water!

CLOCKWISE FROM TOP: casarecce, spaghetti chitarra, manfredi lunghi, taccole, fregola, orechiette, mezzi rigatoni, nodi marini

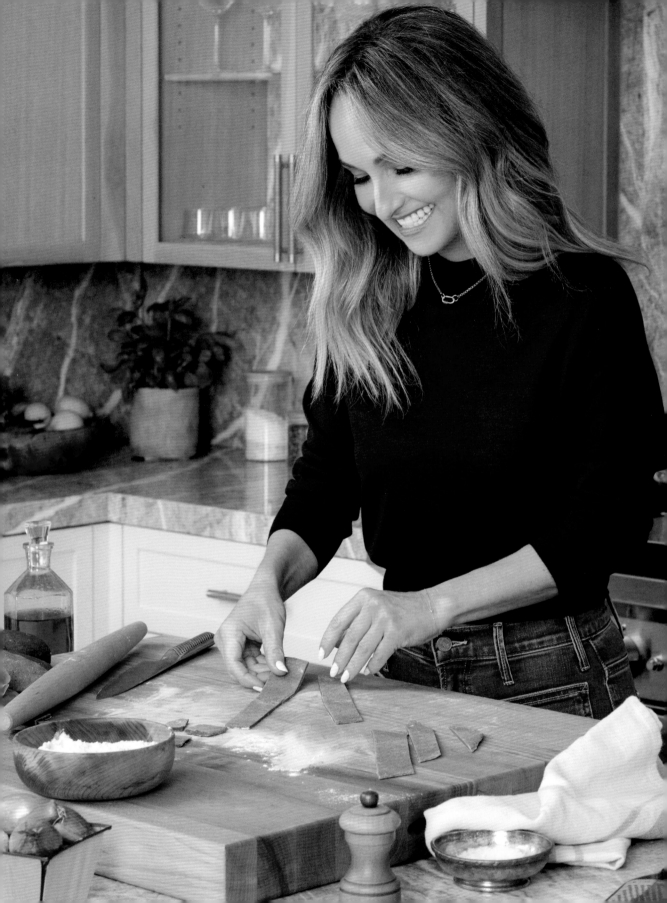

Stracchi WITH Spicy Pomodoro

Stracchi means "rags" in Italian, and these random cuts are the simplest way to shape and serve fresh pasta. I'm not going to pretend I make pasta from scratch all the time, but as a special weekend project, it's something I really enjoy. I don't even bother with a pasta machine, as this soft dough is easy to roll by hand. It's the pasta my family made on Sundays for lasagna, fettuccine, and stuffed pastas like ravioli, and I love the way the bright green pasta contrasts with the sauce. I like the freshly cooked pasta just lightly "stained" with sauce, but if you prefer your pasta more heavily sauced, use a double batch of the pomodoro.

Serves

4

—

1 (5-ounce) package baby spinach (about 6 cups)

1¾ cups all-purpose flour, plus 1 tablespoon for mixing

½ cup semolina flour, plus more for dusting

2 large eggs, at room temperature

3 large egg yolks, at room temperature

2½ cups Calabrian Pomodoro (page 61)

2 tablespoons unsalted butter

½ cup freshly grated Parmigiano-Reggiano cheese

Fill a large bowl with ice and water and set near the sink. Bring a medium pot of generously salted water to a boil. Add the spinach to the boiling water and cook, stirring to submerge the leaves, for just 1 minute. Immediately drain the spinach in a colander, then add to the bowl of ice water.

When the spinach is cool, gather it into a ball and twist to squeeze out as much liquid as possible. Place the spinach in a small blender or food processor and process until completely smooth. If it does not puree completely, add one of the whole eggs and blend again until smooth.

In a large shallow bowl, stir together both flours. Make a well in the center. Add the remaining whole eggs, egg yolks, and spinach puree. Use a fork to break up the eggs, then gradually mix in the flour, drawing it bit by bit from the sides of the bowl until it is all incorporated. As the dough becomes stiffer you may need to use your hands to work in the remaining flour. If the dough seems too sticky, add an extra tablespoon of all-purpose flour; if it is too stiff, add a tiny bit of water until it is soft enough to knead.

Turn the dough onto a work surface and knead until very smooth and pliable, 5 to 6 minutes. Wrap the dough tightly in plastic wrap and set aside to rest for at least 30 minutes.

CONTINUES

Bring a large pot of water to a boil. Pour the pomodoro into a large skillet and bring just to a simmer, then cover and keep warm.

To roll the pasta, dust a work surface and rolling pin lightly with semolina flour. Divide the pasta dough into 4 equal portions. Working with 1 portion at a time, roll the dough as thinly and as evenly as you can, flipping the dough and dusting with a bit more semolina flour only as needed to prevent sticking. (See Hint.) Use a paring knife to cut the dough into random shapes or "rags" about 3 inches square. Scoop the rags onto a sheet pan, dust lightly with semolina flour, and repeat with the remaining dough portions.

Salt the boiling water generously. Add the pasta and cook just until al dente, about 3 minutes. Start checking for doneness after 1 minute, as fresh pasta cooks very quickly. With a skimmer or sieve, transfer the pasta to the skillet with the pomodoro, add the butter and a splash of the pasta water, and cook together over medium heat until the pasta has absorbed some of the sauce. Add a bit more pasta water if the pan seems dry. Serve sprinkled with the Parmigiano.

Spaghetti alla Cabiria

My grandfather Dino De Laurentiis loved food even more than he loved making movies, and when he could combine the two, he was truly in his happy place. On the set of *Le Notti di Cabiria,* a film he produced with writer-director Federico Fellini, he improvised a quick meal for the cast and crew using peperonata, some tomato puree, and chewy spaghetti chitarra. The film went on to win the Academy Award for best foreign film, and I think this flavorful vegetarian pasta is a real winner, too. It's not coated in sauce, just stained, and is a delicious way to repurpose the peperonata you have in the fridge.

Serves
6

3 tablespoons extra-virgin olive oil

2 yellow bell peppers, cored, seeded, and thinly sliced

1 garlic clove, finely chopped

1 cup passata (tomato puree)

½ teaspoon kosher salt, plus more to taste

4 anchovy fillets, finely chopped

2 tablespoons capers, drained

1 cup pitted mixed olives, chopped

1 pound long pasta, such as spaghetti chitarra

2 sprigs fresh basil

2 tablespoons chopped fresh flat-leaf Italian parsley, plus more for serving

In a large deep skillet, heat the oil over medium-high heat. Add the peppers and cook, stirring occasionally, until slightly browned and softened, about 5 minutes. Add the garlic and stir until fragrant and starting to turn golden, another minute or two.

Add the passata, salt, anchovies, capers, olives, and 1 cup water. Bring to a boil, stirring occasionally. Add the basil and parsley. Reduce the heat to low, cover the pan, and simmer gently until the sauce has reduced by about half, about 30 minutes. Add a bit more salt to taste if needed.

While the sauce simmers, bring a large pot of well-salted water to a boil over high heat. Add the pasta and cook, stirring occasionally, until tender but still firm to the bite, 8 to 10 minutes. Reserve ½ cup of the pasta water, then drain the pasta and add it to the skillet with the sauce.

Using tongs, toss the pasta with the sauce to coat, adding the reserved pasta water as needed to loosen the sauce. Serve with a sprinkle of chopped parsley.

Apulian Pasta
with Mussels and Chickpeas

Chickpeas are a major crop in Puglia, so they are a staple in many dishes from this region, including pastas. And because what grows together goes together, cooks in this coastal area often combine the legumes with seafood, as in this unusual and tasty dish. This is known as a classic poor man's dish because it uses inexpensive local ingredients to provide protein in homes where meat didn't appear on the table very often. The good chew of chickpeas and the flavor of mussels make a very frugal pasta that still feels elegant and luxurious.

Serves

6

◆

1 pound orecchiette

2 tablespoons extra-virgin olive oil, plus more for drizzling

1 (15.5-ounce) can chickpeas, drained

1 fennel bulb (stalks removed and fronds reserved for garnish), halved and thinly sliced

2 garlic cloves, finely chopped

1 teaspoon kosher salt

½ teaspoon Calabrian chile paste

1½ teaspoons finely chopped fresh rosemary

1 cup dry white wine

1 (14-ounce) jar yellow datterini tomatoes or 1 pint yellow cherry tomatoes

2 pounds mussels, scrubbed

1 tablespoon fresh lemon juice

½ cup Garlicky Bread Crumbs [page 47]

Bring a large pot of well-salted water to a boil over high heat. Add the pasta and cook until not quite al dente, about 2 minutes less than the package directions. Reserve 1 cup of the pasta water, then drain the pasta.

In a large skillet, heat the oil over medium heat. Add the chickpeas, fennel, garlic, and ½ teaspoon of the salt and cook, stirring often, until the fennel is softened, about 5 minutes. Add the chile paste, 1 teaspoon of the rosemary, and the wine and cook until the wine is reduced by about half, about 4 minutes.

Add the tomatoes and mussels, cover the pan, and cook over medium-high heat until the mussels have just opened, 4 to 5 minutes. Remove from the heat and use a large slotted spoon to transfer the mussels to a bowl.

Remove all but a handful of the mussels from their shells, reserving a few in the shell for decoration, and return all the mussels along with any accumulated juices to the pan. Add the lemon juice and remaining ½ teaspoon salt and cook over medium heat until the pasta is heated through and the liquid is somewhat reduced, 1 to 2 minutes. Add a bit of the pasta water if the pasta looks too dry. Drizzle with a bit more olive oil, sprinkle with the remaining ½ teaspoon rosemary, and toss once more.

Serve sprinkled with the bread crumbs and garnished with the reserved fennel fronds.

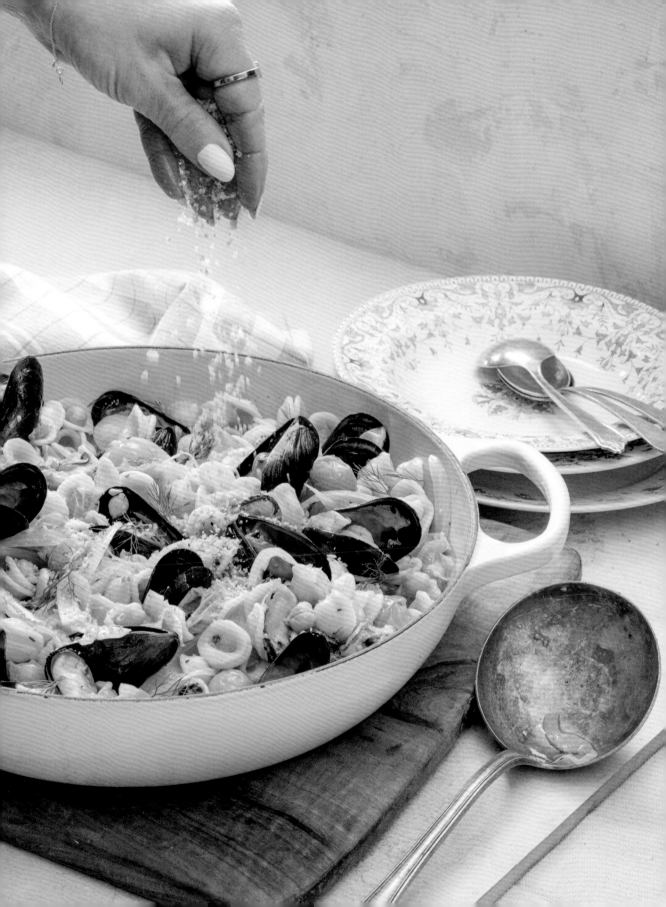

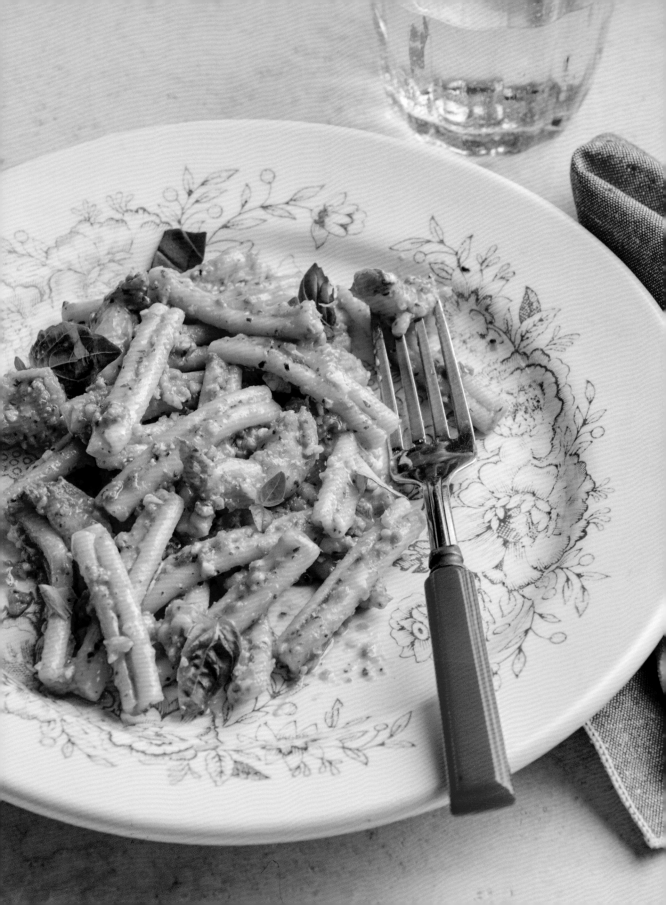

Casarecce with Sicilian Pesto and Shrimp

Frozen shrimp are a great pantry item, and tossed with one of my indispensable condiments, they make for an unexpectedly delicious weeknight meal. As pasta with tomato sauce goes, this one is lighter and fresher because the tomatoes aren't really cooked, just warmed a bit by the hot pasta. My favorite time to make this is in the summer when cherry tomatoes are bursting with flavor. I like it with a short pasta to cradle all the pesto in the nooks and crannies; it won't coat long noodles like spaghetti as well. Even if you have to make the pesto from scratch, you can still pull this dish together in the time it takes to cook the pasta.

Serves
6

◆

1 pound casarecce
or other short pasta

1 tablespoon extra-virgin olive oil

½ pound large shrimp, peeled and
deveined, each cut into
3 or 4 pieces

½ teaspoon kosher salt

2 cups Sicilian Pesto [page 60]

Torn fresh basil leaves, for garnish

Bring a large pot of well-salted water to a boil. Add the pasta and cook until al dente according to the package directions.

While the pasta cooks, in a large sauté pan heat the oil over medium-high heat. When the oil is quite hot, add the shrimp and sprinkle with the salt. Increase the heat to high and cook, stirring frequently, until the shrimp pieces are starting to get some browned spots and are cooked through, about 3 minutes. Stir in the pesto and remove from the heat.

When the pasta is cooked, reserve 1 cup of the pasta water, then drain the pasta and immediately add it to the pan. (See Hint.) Add ¼ cup of the pasta water and toss to combine, scraping the bottom of the pan to loosen any bits of shrimp. If the sauce is too thick, add more pasta water as needed to make a light sauce.

Serve warm or at room temperature, sprinkled with the basil leaves.

HINT HINT ◆ If your pan isn't large enough to hold all the pasta, transfer it to a large serving bowl after draining. Use ¼ cup of the pasta water to loosen the sauce, then add it to the pasta and toss to coat.

Ziti with Roasted Garlic and Arugula Pesto

I've never loved the sharp bite of raw garlic you get with most pestos; when you substitute mellow roasted garlic for raw, you can use a lot more—a whole head in this instance—for a deep, rich flavor and none of the sharpness. Here I've paired the garlic with arugula and pistachios for a dreamy green sauce that contrasts beautifully with simple pan-roasted tomatoes.

Serves
6

◆

1 head garlic

½ cup plus 3 tablespoons extra-virgin olive oil

¾ teaspoon kosher salt

1 pound ziti corti or other short pasta

3 cups baby arugula

¼ cup salted roasted pistachios, plus more for garnish

¼ teaspoon freshly ground black pepper

½ cup freshly grated Parmigiano-Reggiano cheese

2 teaspoons fresh lemon juice

1 pint cherry tomatoes

¼ teaspoon flaky salt (or use additional kosher salt)

Grated zest of 1 small lemon, for garnish

Preheat the oven to 475°F.

Cut the garlic head in half horizontally and place on a sheet of foil. Drizzle the cut surfaces with 1 tablespoon of the oil and sprinkle with ¼ teaspoon of the kosher salt. Fold the foil up and around the garlic, enclosing it completely. Place on a baking sheet and roast until very soft, about 20 minutes.

Bring a large pot of well-salted water to a boil. Add the pasta and cook until al dente according to the package directions. Reserve 1 cup of the pasta water, then drain the pasta and return to the pasta pot.

Meanwhile, in a food processor, combine the roasted garlic, arugula, pistachios, the remaining ½ teaspoon kosher salt, and the pepper in a food processor. Process until coarsely ground. With the motor running, stream in ½ cup oil until smooth. Add the cheese and lemon juice and pulse two or three times to combine. Set the arugula pesto aside.

In a medium skillet, heat the remaining 2 tablespoons oil over medium heat. (See Hint.) Add the tomatoes and pan-roast, shaking every few minutes, until they start to blister, about 5 minutes. Sprinkle with the flaky salt.

Add the arugula pesto and about ½ cup of the pasta water to the pasta pot. Toss over medium-high heat until the pasta is well sauced and warmed through.

Serve topped with the tomatoes, a few chopped pistachios, and a bit of lemon zest.

HINT HINT ◆ If you prefer, you can roast the tomatoes on the sheet pan along with the garlic, cooking them for about 6 minutes, or until they are just starting to collapse.

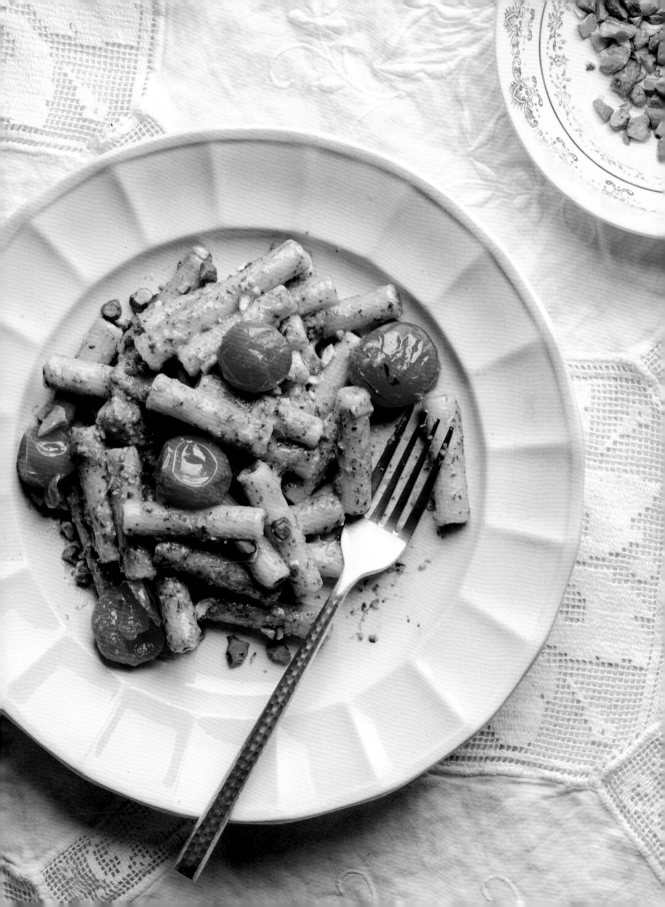

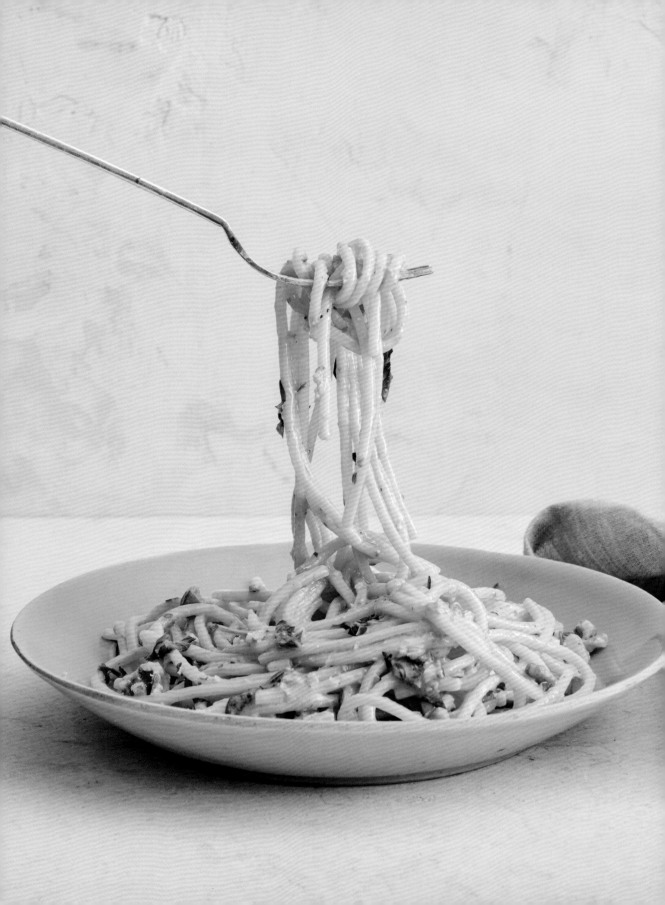

Anchovy Pasta
WITH Walnuts

There are anchovies in quite a few of the recipes in this book, but in most cases, they play a supporting role. Here they are front and center, elevating a few pantry ingredients to something worthy of company. It's actually a play on aglio e olio as it's made on the Amalfi Coast, where seafood of all kinds features often in the pasta dishes. The anchovies and colatura add complexity and depth to an otherwise simple dish; just be sure to mash them up really well in the oil. I added arugula because I am a nut when it comes to greens—I need some in every meal—and it makes this a one-pot meal.

Serves
6

◆

1 pound long pasta, such as spaghetti chitarra or linguine

1 teaspoon Calabrian chile paste, or to taste

2 anchovy fillets, finely chopped

½ teaspoon colatura (or an additional anchovy)

½ cup extra-virgin olive oil

1 cup freshly grated Parmigiano-Reggiano cheese

½ cup walnuts, toasted and coarsely chopped

½ cup fresh mint leaves, coarsely chopped

2 cups baby arugula

Bring a large pot of well-salted water to a boil over high heat. Add the pasta and cook until al dente according to the package directions. Reserve 1 cup of the pasta water, then drain the pasta well.

In a large bowl, whisk together the chile paste, anchovies, colatura, and oil. Add the pasta, top with the grated cheese, and toss well, adding the pasta water as needed to create a sauce. Add the walnuts, mint, and arugula, toss well, and serve.

Orecchiette WITH Almond Pesto AND Broccoli Rabe

Here's a meatless pasta that should be in everyone's repertoire. It has so many different tastes and textures that no one will miss the meat. It's equally good warm or at room temperature and works both as a main and a side dish. The almonds add depth and richness without tasting almond-y; you just get the roasty richness. If you are a fan of orecchiette with sausage and broccoli rabe, you should give this one a try; it has that same comforting taste and feeling. And if you don't love broccoli rabe, go ahead and substitute milder tasting broccolini or regular broccoli.

Serves
6

—

2 bunches broccoli rabe

½ cup unsalted roasted almonds

2 cups (packed) fresh basil leaves

¾ cup extra-virgin olive oil

1 teaspoon kosher salt

1 cup freshly grated Parmigiano-Reggiano cheese, plus more for serving

½ pound smoked mozzarella cheese, cut into ⅓-inch dice

1 pound orecchiette

Bring a large pot of well-salted water to a boil. Add the broccoli rabe and cook for 4 minutes, then use tongs to transfer to a colander, leaving the water in the pot. When cool enough to handle, cut the broccoli rabe into 1-inch pieces.

In a food processor, pulse the almonds 5 or 6 times until finely chopped. Add the basil, oil, and ½ teaspoon salt and puree until almost smooth.

Pour the mixture into a large bowl. Add the Parmigiano, broccoli rabe, and mozzarella and toss well to combine.

Bring the water in the broccoli rabe pot back to a boil and add the orecchiette. Cook until al dente according to the package directions. Using a skimmer or large slotted spoon, transfer the pasta directly into the bowl with the pesto. Add ½ cup of the pasta water and the remaining ½ teaspoon salt and toss until the pasta is well coated with the sauce.

Top with grated Parmigiano and serve warm or at room temperature.

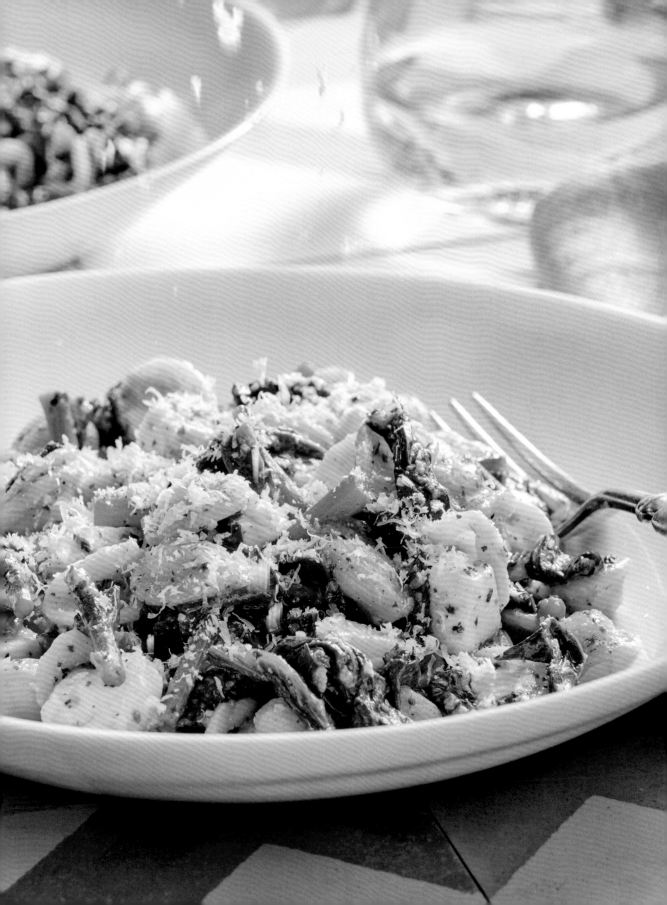

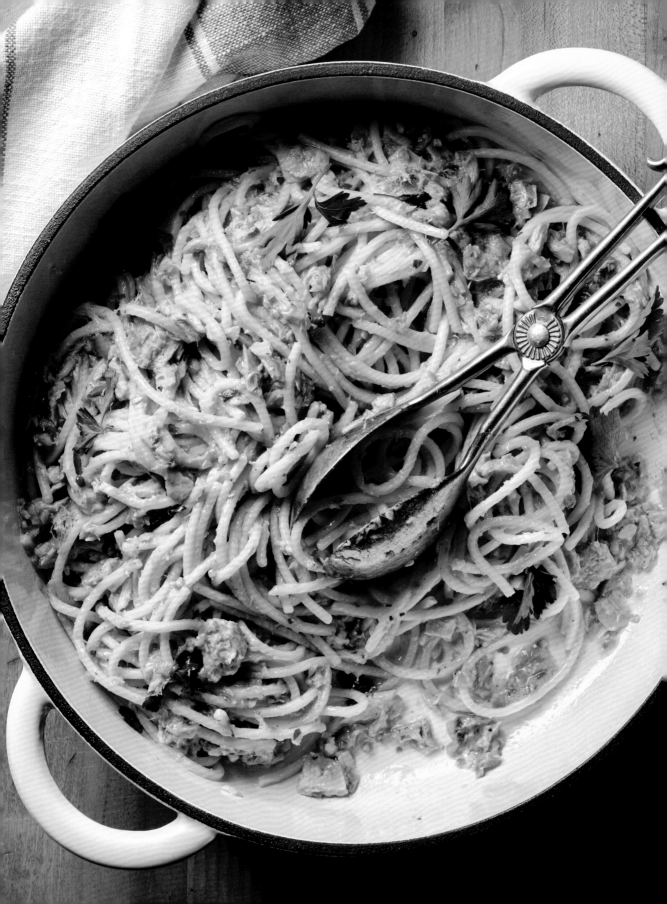

Pantry Pasta
WITH **Tuna** AND **Olives**

As kids, we had this pasta all the time, a homey dish that was a fixture in my mother's repertoire. It will be familiar to anyone who grew up in an Italian household because it's cheap, fast, and easy. But don't let that accessibility fool you; this is deeply flavorful and comforting, and you won't even need to shop to make it if your pantry is up to date. If you like, add some vegetables—such as peas or chopped broccoli florets, or a green like kale or chard—along with the tuna and toss together for 2 to 3 minutes.

Serves
6

❖

1 pound spaghetti chitarra

2 tablespoons extra-virgin olive oil

2 garlic cloves, smashed and peeled

2 anchovy fillets

¼ teaspoon red pepper flakes (optional)

¾ cup Green Olive Relish (page 55) or store-bought green olive tapenade

2 (5-ounce) cans tuna packed in olive oil, drained

½ cup freshly grated pecorino cheese, plus more for serving

¼ cup fresh flat-leaf Italian parsley leaves or chopped arugula

Grated lemon zest (optional) for garnish

Bring a large pot of well-salted water to a boil over high heat. Add the pasta and cook until not quite al dente, about 2 minutes less than the package directions.

Meanwhile, heat a large skillet over medium heat. Add the oil, garlic, and anchovies and cook until the garlic is aromatic and beginning to brown, about 30 seconds. Add the pepper flakes (if using), olive relish, and tuna. Remove the pan from the heat. Stir gently to combine, being careful not to break up the tuna too finely.

When the pasta is ready, add ½ cup of the pasta water to the skillet with the tuna mixture and return it to medium heat. Using tongs, transfer the pasta from the water directly to the skillet. Sprinkle the pasta with the pecorino and toss well until the sauce coats the pasta strands. Add more pasta water if the sauce is too dry. Stir in the parsley and top with more pecorino cheese or lemon zest if desired.

Pasta alla Zozzona

This one is as much fun to say as it is to eat. *Zozzona* means "dirty" in the sense that it is a big mess, an exuberant mash-up of Amatriciana, carbonara, alla gricia, and cacio e pepe, the four classic pasta dishes of Rome. This is usually made with generous amounts of pancetta, cheese, *and* sweet Italian sausage on top of the egg yolks, which is just too rich for my palate. But even with my nods to moderation—tweaking the amount of pancetta and subbing in lighter turkey sausage for pork sausage—I think you'll agree this is still a very decadent dish!

Serves
6 TO 8

4 large egg yolks

1 cup freshly grated Parmigiano-Reggiano cheese, plus more (optional) for serving

½ cup freshly grated pecorino cheese

2 ounces diced pancetta

2 tablespoons extra-virgin olive oil

1 pound sweet Italian turkey or chicken sausage, casings removed

2 shallots, diced

3 garlic cloves, smashed and peeled

¼ teaspoon kosher salt

2 cups passata (tomato puree)

1 teaspoon freshly ground black pepper

1 teaspoon Calabrian chile paste

1 pound short pasta, such as nodi marini or fusilli

In a small bowl, combine the egg yolks and the Parmigiano and pecorino. Stir together with a rubber spatula. Set aside.

In a large skillet, heat the oil over medium heat. Add the pancetta and cook until browned and crisp, about 5 minutes.

Use a slotted spoon to transfer the pancetta to a paper towel to drain, then pour out all but about 1 tablespoon of the fat in the pan. Add the sausage to the skillet, breaking it into small pieces with the back of a spoon, and cook until it is lightly browned and cooked through, about 7 minutes.

Add the shallots, garlic, and salt to the pan and cook until soft and fragrant, another 3 minutes. Stir in the passata, pepper, and chile paste and bring the sauce to a simmer. Cook for 10 minutes to allow the flavors to marry.

While the sauce cooks, bring a large pot of well-salted water to a boil over high heat. Add the pasta and cook until not quite al dente, about 2 minutes less than the package directions. Reserve 1 cup of the pasta water, then drain the pasta.

Add the cooked pasta to the sauce along with ½ cup pasta water. Toss and stir over medium-high heat to coat the pasta in the sauce and finish cooking the pasta. Add up to ¼ cup more pasta water if the sauce gets too thick.

Temper the egg yolk/cheese mixture with ¼ cup pasta water, stirring constantly to prevent scrambling. When the pasta is al dente and coated in the sauce, remove the pan from the heat. Quickly stir in the egg yolk mixture, tossing and stirring until the sauce is creamy and glossy and clings to the pasta. Serve with additional Parmigiano if desired.

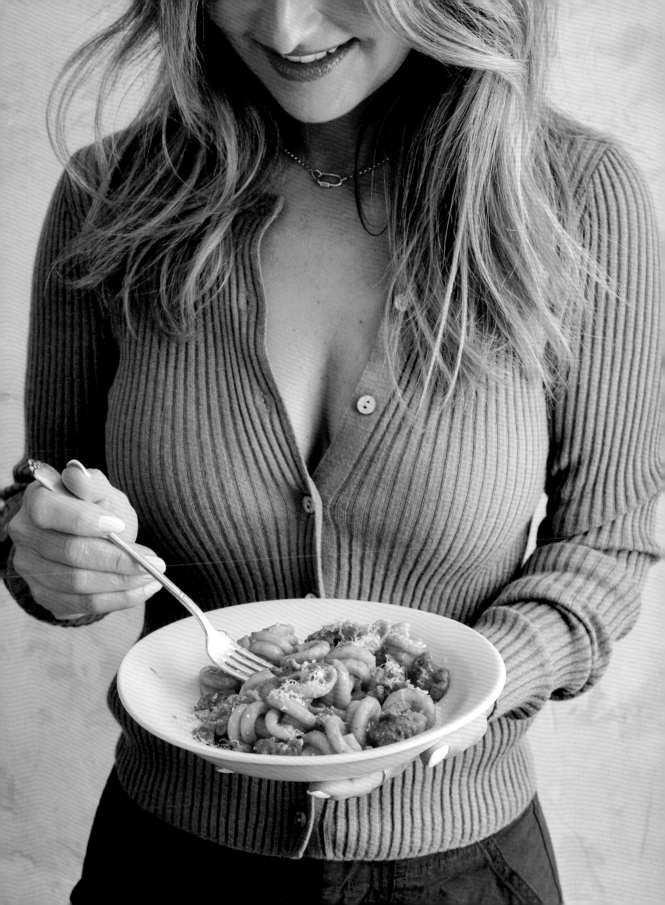

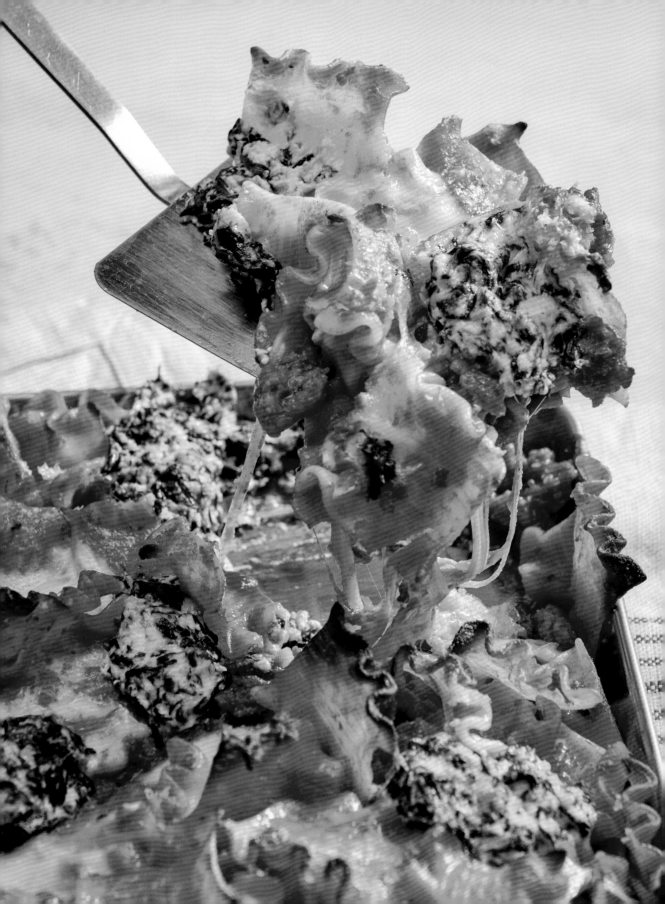

Layerless Sheet Pan Lasagna

This was a viral sensation when I first introduced it on Giadzy, and it's now my favorite way to serve a group. I came up with it as a way to double down on the part of the lasagna I like best—the crispy frilly edges—and now I've lightened it up a bit for a *slightly* less indulgent version.

Serves
6 TO 8
(SEE HINT)

4 tablespoons extra-virgin olive oil

1 garlic clove, chopped

½ teaspoon red pepper flakes

1 (5-ounce) package baby spinach (about 6 cups)

½ teaspoon kosher salt

1 cup part-skim ricotta cheese

1 pound spicy chicken sausage, casings removed

1 red onion, diced

1 pound taccole pasta or lasagne noodles broken into 2-inch pieces

4 cups Simple Tomato Sauce (page 63) or Calabrian Pomodoro (page 61)

1 pound firm (low-moisture) mozzarella cheese, half diced, half sliced

1 cup freshly grated Parmigiano-Reggiano cheese

HINT HINT ◆ For a weeknight dinner, halve the ingredients and make it on a quarter-sheet pan or in a 9 × 13-inch lasagna pan.

Preheat the oven to 425°F. Oil a sheet pan with 1 tablespoon of the olive oil and set aside.

Heat a large skillet over medium heat. Add 1 tablespoon oil, the garlic, and the pepper flakes and cook, stirring often, until fragrant, about 1 minute. Add the spinach and salt and cook until wilted, stirring frequently, another minute or two. Remove the spinach mixture to a sieve and press with the back of a spoon to release as much liquid as possible. Chop the spinach fairly finely. Place the spinach in a medium bowl and stir in the ricotta.

Wipe out the skillet and return it to medium heat. Add the remaining 2 tablespoons oil and the sausage. Cook the sausage without moving it until the underside is browned, about 3 minutes. Using a wooden spoon, break the sausage into bite-size pieces. Continue to cook, stirring often, until the sausage is lightly browned on all sides, 4 to 5 minutes. Add the onion and cook until it is fragrant and beginning to soften, another 3 minutes. Remove from the heat.

Meanwhile, bring a large pot of well-salted water to a boil over high heat. Add the pasta and cook for 4 minutes, stirring often to avoid clumping. Reserve ½ cup of the pasta water, then drain the pasta well.

Add the sauce and pasta water to the skillet with the sausage and onion and mix well. Stir in the diced mozzarella, the pasta, and ½ cup of the Parmigiano.

Spread the mixture on the prepared sheet pan. Dollop with the ricotta-spinach mixture and tuck the sliced mozzarella in among the noodles. Sprinkle with the remaining ½ cup Parmigiano. Bake until lightly browned, about 25 minutes.

Let rest for 5 minutes before cutting into squares and serving.

Cavatelli WITH Eggplant AND Smoked Mozzarella

Pasta alla Norma is a fabled Sicilian dish that is especially popular for those in search of a hearty vegetarian pasta option. In conventional versions, the eggplant is fried to give it a meat-like chew and rich flavor; I wanted to see if I could make it a little lighter and brighter, so I roasted the eggplant instead of frying it and paired it with a quickly cooked fresh tomato sauce that stains rather than coats the pasta. To amplify the flavor even further, I have substituted smoked mozzarella for the usual ricotta salata, as I love the smokier notes with the roasted eggplant. It's simple but sumptuous.

Serves
6

❧

2 medium eggplants
(about 1½ pounds in total)

5 tablespoons extra-virgin olive oil

3½ teaspoons kosher salt,
plus more to taste

3 garlic cloves,
smashed and peeled

1½ pounds Campari or stem
tomatoes, cut into large dice

¼ cup (lightly packed) chopped
fresh basil, plus torn leaves
for garnish

1 pound short pasta, such as
cavatelli or orecchiette

5 ounces smoked mozzarella
cheese cut into ½-inch dice
(about 1¼ cups)

Position a rack in the upper third of the oven and preheat the oven to 450°F. Line a sheet pan with parchment paper.

Trim the stem end of the eggplants, then cut into irregular 1-inch chunks. Spread the eggplant pieces on the lined pan and drizzle with 2 tablespoons of the oil. Sprinkle with 2 teaspoons of the salt, toss, and roast on the top rack of the oven until the eggplant has some deep brown spots but the pieces still hold their shape, 20 to 25 minutes, tossing every 10 minutes.

Meanwhile, in a large skillet, heat the remaining 3 tablespoons oil over medium heat. Add the garlic and cook until fragrant and lightly browned, about 3 minutes. Discard the garlic, then add the tomatoes and cook, stirring often, until the tomato pieces are becoming soft and juicy, about 6 minutes. Stir in the basil and remaining 1½ teaspoons salt and remove from the heat.

Bring a large pot of well-salted water to a boil. Add the pasta and cook until not quite al dente, about 2 minutes less than the package directions. Using a large slotted spoon, scoop the pasta directly into the skillet with the tomato sauce. Add ¼ cup of the pasta water and ¾ cup of the mozzarella.

Cook the pasta with the sauce over medium-low heat, stirring constantly, until the sauce is creamy and the pasta is cooked through. Add pasta water as needed to maintain a loose sauce. Add the eggplant, cook for another minute to heat through, and add a bit more salt to taste.

Serve sprinkled with the remaining ½ cup mozzarella and the torn basil leaves.

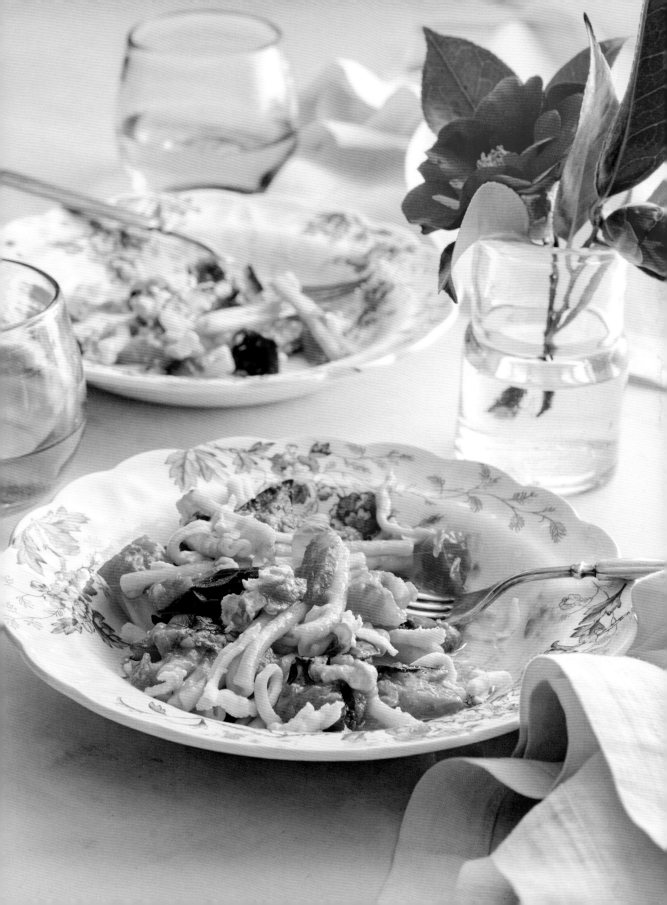

Spaghetti Chitarra
with Zucchini, Lemon, and Shrimp

Can you improve on perfection? This recipe has been revered for generations—I remember my grandfather raving about it when he came back from a vacation on the Amalfi Coast. It's the specialty of a restaurant called Lo Scoglio in the town of Nerano, south of Positano, and tourists line up for the house specialty, pasta combined with simple shallow-fried zucchini. I've put my own spin on it by adding extra lemon and shrimp for protein, turning it into a one-pan meal. Timing is everything here: You need to get the pasta going before you make the zucchini puree. Take your time cooking the zucchini. Yes, the zucchini is fried, but let's remember, these are not potato chips or French fries, and the process makes a somewhat bland vegetable super tasty, velvety, and buttery instead of watery and mushy.

Serves

4

◆

½ pound large shrimp, peeled and deveined

1 tablespoon extra-virgin olive oil

Grated zest and juice of 1 small lemon, plus additional zest for serving

1½ teaspoons kosher salt, plus more for pureeing

½ teaspoon red pepper flakes

1 cup olive oil, for frying

2 garlic cloves, smashed and peeled

3 medium zucchini, sliced ¼ inch thick

1 pound spaghetti chitarra

Bring a large pot of well-salted water to a boil for the pasta.

In a bowl, combine the shrimp, extra-virgin olive oil, lemon zest and juice, ½ teaspoon of the salt, and the pepper flakes. Toss to coat the shrimp well.

Line a large plate with paper towels and set near the stove. In a large skillet, heat the 1 cup olive oil and garlic together over medium heat until the oil is very hot and the garlic is lightly browned, about 2 minutes. Discard the garlic and increase the heat to medium-high. When the oil is very hot, add half the zucchini and fry until golden, about 10 minutes, turning to brown the slices on both sides. Make sure the pan and oil are quite hot before you add the zucchini; you want it to fry, not steam. Use a slotted spoon to transfer the zucchini to the paper towels to drain. Sprinkle with ½ teaspoon salt. Add the remaining zucchini to the pan and fry as you did the first batch.

While the zucchini cooks, add the pasta to the boiling water and cook until not quite al dente, about 2 minutes less than the package directions. Reserve 2 cups of the pasta water, then drain the pasta and set aside.

Transfer half the fried zucchini to a blender and add 1 tablespoon of oil (you can use the oil you fried the zucchini in if it is not too dark), the basil leaves, the Parmigiano, and 1 cup pasta water. Season with a pinch of salt and puree until smooth. Set aside.

Pour out the hot frying oil but don't wipe out the skillet. Add the shrimp in a single layer and cook until just beginning to brown at the edges, about 90 seconds. Turn the shrimp and cook for another 60 seconds on the second side. You don't want them to cook through, just get some nice golden color. Remove from the heat and use kitchen shears to cut each shrimp into 3 or 4 pieces, returning the pieces to the skillet.

Add the pureed zucchini to the pan with the shrimp along with the remaining fried zucchini, black pepper (if using), and 1 cup pasta water. Use tongs to transfer the pasta directly from the pot to the skillet, add the butter (if using), and toss over medium heat until the sauce is silky. Serve topped with a bit more lemon zest, Parmigiano, and basil.

10 large fresh basil leaves, torn, plus more for serving

Freshly ground black pepper (optional)

1 cup freshly grated Parmigiano-Reggiano cheese, plus more for serving

2 tablespoons unsalted butter (optional)

Creamy Pasta
WITH **Asparagus**

It's always a smart idea to have a few vegetarian pasta recipes in your repertoire, and this one is right up my alley, with my favorite fennel, luxurious asparagus, a light creamy sauce, and a hint of lemon to bring it all together. To keep the green theme going, I add some chopped pistachios for crunch.

Serves

6

◆

1 pound asparagus, bottom inch trimmed

1 pound spaghetti or other long pasta

3 tablespoons extra-virgin olive oil, plus more for drizzling

2 shallots, diced

1 medium fennel bulb (stalks removed), very thinly sliced crosswise

½ teaspoon Calabrian chile paste

1¼ teaspoons kosher salt

1 cup ricotta cheese, preferably whole-milk

Grated zest and juice of 1 lemon

½ cup freshly grated Parmigiano-Reggiano cheese

¼ cup chopped salted roasted pistachios

Freshly ground black pepper (optional)

Bring a large pot of well-salted water to a boil over medium-high heat.

While the water heats, cut off the top 3 inches of each asparagus spear and set aside. Cut the remaining stalks into ½-inch pieces.

Add the pasta to the water and stir to prevent sticking. Cook until just al dente, according to the package directions.

While the pasta is cooking, in a large skillet, heat the oil over medium-high heat. Add the shallots, fennel, chile paste, and ½ teaspoon of the salt. Cook, stirring often, until the fennel has softened and is beginning to brown lightly, 3 to 4 minutes. Add all the asparagus and the remaining ¾ teaspoon salt and cook, stirring occasionally, until the asparagus is tender, 2 to 4 minutes. Stir in the ricotta and, using a ladle, add enough pasta water to make a creamy sauce. Stir in the lemon zest and juice.

Using tongs, add the pasta directly from the water to the skillet and sprinkle with the Parmigiano. Stir to combine and toss to coat the pasta, adding pasta water as needed if the mixture seems too dry. Serve drizzled with more olive oil, the pistachios, and a few grinds of pepper (if using).

Pasta Assassina

Forget everything you know about making pasta here: The pasta is cooked in a nearly dry pan to start, and you want to bring the strands right to the edge of burning to get some strong caramelization on the bottom of the pan. Once you've got that caramelization going, you cook it more like a risotto than a pasta, adding ladlesful of tomato-tinged water a bit at a time until the pasta is tender. You need to watch the pasta carefully (don't walk away from it!), but the result is *so* full of flavor. Although it is not traditional (and optional for those who haven't yet boarded the tinned fish train), I like to add canned sardines just before plating for a bit of protein—and all those Super-Italian nutrients. Oh, and the name? Its origins are a bit unclear, but I do know that this pasta slays every time!

Serves
3 TO 4

¼ cup tomato paste

1 teaspoon kosher salt

¼ cup extra-virgin olive oil, plus more for drizzling

4 garlic cloves, smashed and peeled

1 teaspoon Calabrian chile paste

1 cup passata (tomato puree)

8 ounces spaghetti

2 tins boneless sardines (optional)

Finely chopped fresh flat-leaf Italian parsley, for serving

¼ cup freshly grated pecorino cheese

In a saucepan, bring 3 cups water to a boil. Stir in the tomato paste and salt and keep warm over very low heat.

In a large sauté pan, warm the oil, garlic, and chile paste over medium-high heat until the chiles are sizzling and the garlic is lightly browned, about 4 minutes. Discard the garlic. Add the passata to the pan and cook for 2 minutes to thicken slightly, then add the raw pasta. Turn the pasta strands to coat, then spread them in the pan, trying to bring as many of the strands into contact with the bottom of the pan as possible. Cook without stirring until the pasta starts to caramelize, about 2 minutes. Toss, spread out again, and cook for another 2 minutes.

Add about 1 cup of the warm tomato water to the pan and simmer the pasta until most of the liquid has been absorbed. As the pasta absorbs the water, the oil will begin to sizzle and fry the pasta, which is what you want. Toss the pasta, scraping up the browned bits from the bottom of the pan and repeat the process two more times. When you add the final cup of tomato water, add the sardines to the pan (if using). Stir gently to cover with the sauce and heat through.

Serve garnished with a bit of parsley, the pecorino, and a drizzle of olive oil.

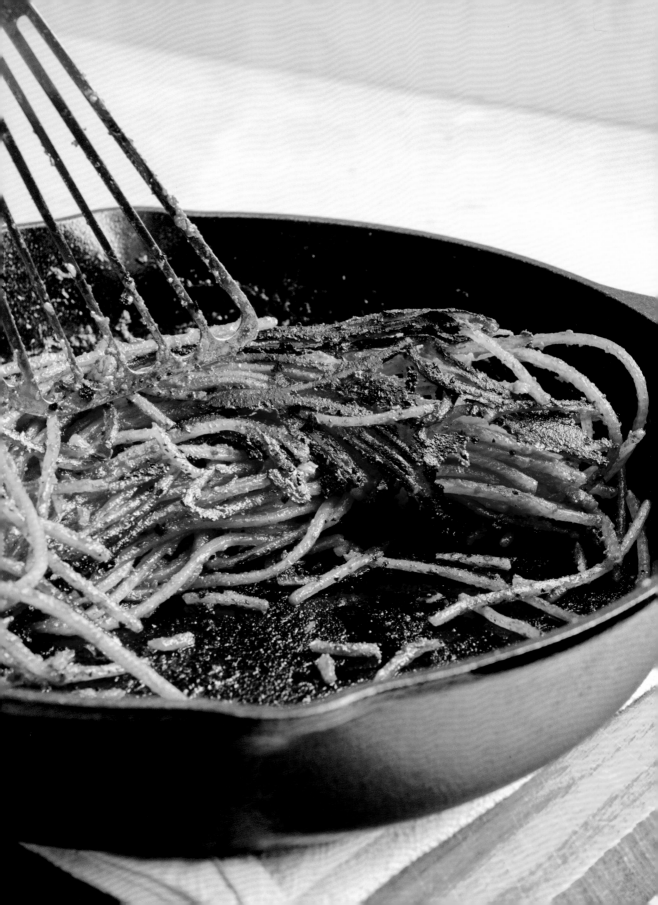

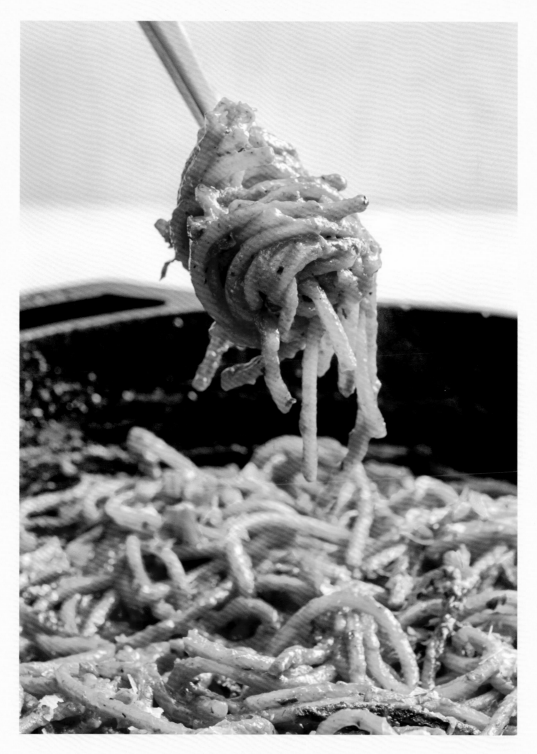

PASTA ASSASSINA ◆ PAGE 141

Baked Pasta WITH Turkey AND Broccoli Rabe Meatballs

Baked pastas are one of the easiest ways to serve a crowd, with a tempting browned crust of gooey cheese that brings everyone to the table. But let's not kid ourselves, they also tend to be calorically dense and higher in fat than is good for us on a regular basis. Not so with this version, which is loaded with good-for-you turkey meatballs dotted with broccoli rabe, and a lot less cheese than your typical baked ziti or lasagna. Made with only half a pound of pasta, it's also a lower-carb alternative that still feels very rich and indulgent.

Serves

6 TO 8

◆

½ bunch broccoli rabe
(about 4 ounces before trimming)

½ pound short pasta

1 pound ground turkey

1 large egg

½ small red onion, grated

½ cup Garlicky Bread Crumbs
(page 47)

⅔ cup plus ¼ cup freshly grated
pecorino cheese

1 teaspoon grated lemon zest

½ teaspoon kosher salt

2 tablespoons extra-virgin olive oil

3 cups Simple Tomato Sauce
(page 63) or Calabrian Pomodoro
(page 61)

1 pound mozzarella cheese,
half grated, half thinly sliced

Preheat the oven to 450°F.

Bring a large pot of well-salted water to a boil. Trim the tough lower stems from the broccoli rabe and reserve for another use. Add the tender leaves and florets to the boiling water and cook for 2 minutes after the water returns to a boil. Use tongs to transfer the greens to a colander and drain very well.

Add the pasta to the same pot and cook until not quite al dente, about 2 minutes less than the package directions. Reserve ½ cup of the pasta water, then drain the pasta and transfer to a large bowl.

While the pasta cooks, in another large bowl, combine the turkey, egg, onion, bread crumbs, ⅔ cup of the pecorino, the lemon zest, and the salt. Wrap the broccoli rabe in a kitchen towel and press to squeeze out as much water as possible. Chop the broccoli rabe finely (you will have about ½ packed cup) and add to the bowl.

With your hands or a rubber spatula, work the meatball mixture together just until blended. Roll the mixture into balls about 1½ inches in diameter; you should have about 24 meatballs.

In a large sauté pan (see Hint), heat the oil over medium heat. Add the meatballs and cook until firm and lightly browned all over, 6 to 8 minutes, shaking the pan and turning the meatballs often. Add the sauce to the pan and bring to a boil, using a wooden spoon to scrape up any browned bits from the bottom of the pan. Simmer the meatballs in the sauce until cooked through, about 5 minutes.

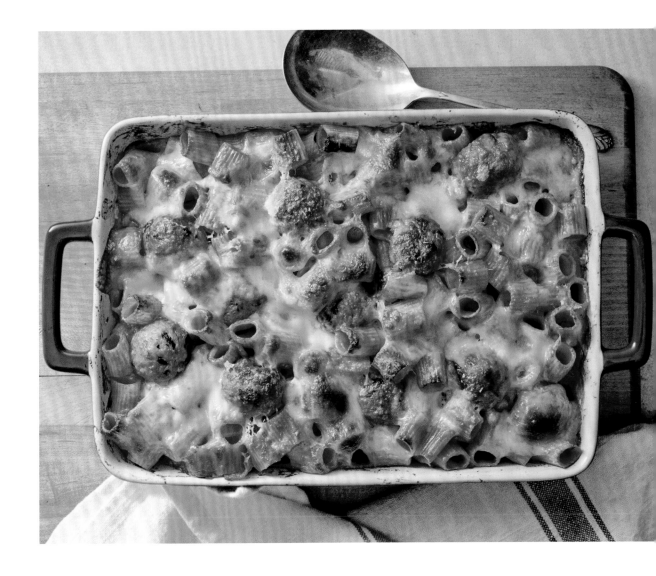

HINT HINT ◆ If you don't have a large sauté pan, you may need to brown the meatballs in two batches. If so, add the pomodoro to the pan with the second batch of meatballs, then return the first batch of meatballs to the pan and simmer them all together. Combine the sauce and the meatballs with the pasta in a large bowl before layering into the baking dish.

Pour the sauce and meatballs over the pasta and gently combine with a rubber spatula. If the mixture doesn't look saucy enough, add a bit of pasta water, 2 tablespoons at a time.

Pour half the pasta and meatball mixture into a 9 × 13-inch baking dish and top with the grated mozzarella. Spread the remaining pasta and meatballs in the dish and arrange the sliced mozzarella on top. Sprinkle with the remaining ¼ cup pecorino.

Bake until the cheese is bubbling and the top is golden, about 20 minutes. Let the pasta rest for at least 10 minutes before serving.

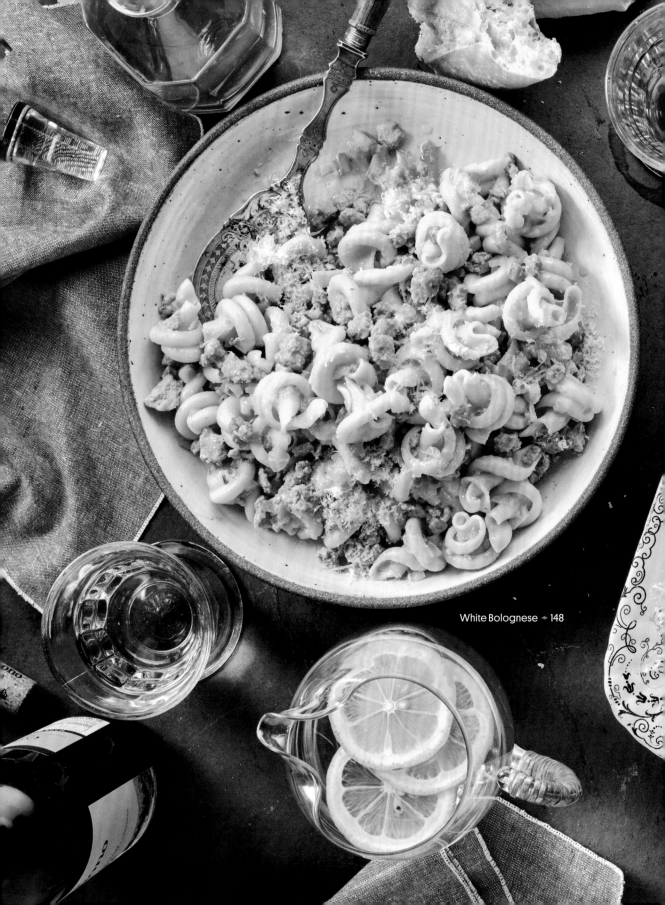

White Bolognese • 148

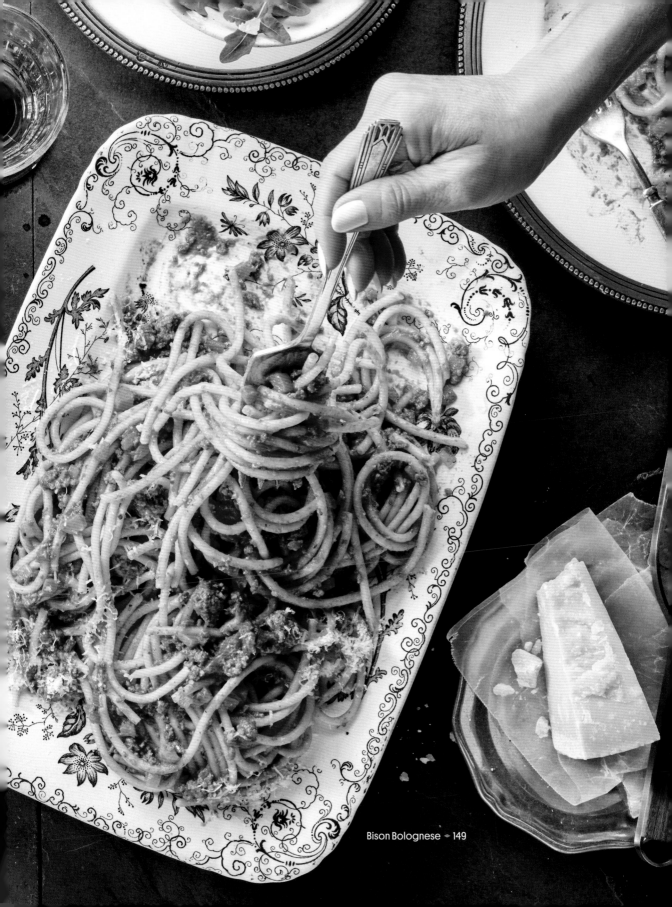

Bison Bolognese ◆ 149

White Bolognese

When I make pasta in the cooler months, I go for something decadent and rib-sticking, often with a meaty element. In the North of Italy you will find quite a few white Bolognese sauces and because they contain no tomato sauce to mask the flavor of meat, they are both lighter and somehow more indulgent. This has the creaminess of an alfredo sauce without the fat and more protein. It's just the thing for a lazy winter afternoon.

Serves
6

1 tablespoon extra-virgin olive oil

4 ounces diced pancetta

1 pound ground dark-meat turkey

1 teaspoon kosher salt

1 carrot, peeled and finely diced

1 fennel bulb (stalks removed), finely diced

½ onion, finely diced

2 garlic cloves, smashed and peeled

½ cup dry white wine

1 cup low-sodium chicken broth

2-inch piece Parmigiano-Reggiano rind

2 fresh basil sprigs

1 cup whole milk

1 pound short pasta, such as nodi marini

1 cup freshly grated Parmigiano-Reggiano cheese, plus more (optional) for serving

Heat a Dutch oven or large sauté pan over medium heat. Add the oil and pancetta and cook, stirring often, until the pancetta is lightly browned and starting to crisp, 7 to 8 minutes. Add the turkey and ½ teaspoon of the salt. Cook, breaking apart the turkey with the back of a wooden spoon, until the turkey is almost fully cooked and a little pink remains, about 6 minutes. Add the carrot, fennel, onion, garlic, and the remaining ½ teaspoon salt. Cook, stirring occasionally, until the vegetables are fragrant and beginning to soften, another 5 minutes. Stir in the wine and simmer until almost fully reduced, about 7 minutes. Add the chicken broth, Parmigiano rind, and basil sprigs and simmer until the mixture is reduced by half, 10 to 12 minutes. Stir in the milk and simmer until slightly reduced, 5 to 6 minutes longer. Remove and discard the rind and basil sprigs.

Meanwhile, bring a large pot of well-salted water to a boil. Add the pasta and cook until not quite al dente, about 2 minutes less than the package directions. Use a spider strainer or slotted spoon to scoop the pasta directly into the sauce. Add ½ cup of the pasta water to the pan, then sprinkle with the Parmigiano and toss to coat every strand. Simmer, adding more pasta water if the sauce seems too dry, until the pasta is al dente and the sauce lightly clings to the pasta, another 2 to 3 minutes.

Serve with more Parmigiano if desired.

Bison Bolognese

I've created a lot of Bolognese recipes in my day and they are incredibly popular in most houses, including mine. Bison is a meat I've been interested in for a while because it is sustainably and responsibly raised, and it's much leaner than most cuts of beef so it cooks quickly. Put the pasta on to boil as the sauce simmers, pull together a salad or a side, and you will have a hearty meal on the table in about 40 minutes.

Serves
6

---

3 tablespoons extra-virgin olive oil, plus more for drizzling

1 pound ground bison

½ red onion, finely chopped

1 medium carrot, peeled and finely diced

2 garlic cloves, smashed and peeled

2 teaspoons kosher salt

1 cup dry white wine

1 (28-ounce) can whole peeled plum tomatoes, undrained

3-inch piece Parmigiano-Reggiano rind

2 stalks fresh basil

1 pound spaghetti or pappardelle

1 cup freshly grated Parmigiano-Reggiano cheese, plus more for serving

2 tablespoons unsalted butter

In a medium Dutch oven, heat the oil over medium-high heat. Add the bison and cook, breaking the meat into small pieces with a wooden spoon, until the meat is lightly browned, about 8 minutes. Stir in the onion, carrot, garlic, and 1 teaspoon of the salt and cook until the vegetables are softened, 3 or 4 minutes.

Add the wine to the pan and stir, scraping up the browned bits from the bottom of the pan. Reduce the heat and simmer until the wine is almost completely reduced, about 5 minutes. Add the tomatoes and their juices, crushing the tomatoes with your hands, and stir well. Season with the remaining 1 teaspoon salt, then nestle the Parmigiano rind and basil into the liquid.

Bring the sauce to a simmer over medium heat, then reduce the heat and continue simmering, stirring occasionally, until there is a ring of cooked tomato around the sides of the pan and the sauce is slightly thickened, about 25 minutes.

While the sauce cooks, bring a large pot of well-salted water to a boil over high heat. Add the pasta and cook until not quite al dente, about 2 minutes less than the package directions.

Use tongs to transfer the pasta directly into the sauce, then add the grated Parmigiano and the butter. Toss the pasta very well, thinning the sauce with pasta water as needed to coat every strand.

Serve the pasta drizzled with a bit of olive oil and a sprinkle of Parmigiano.

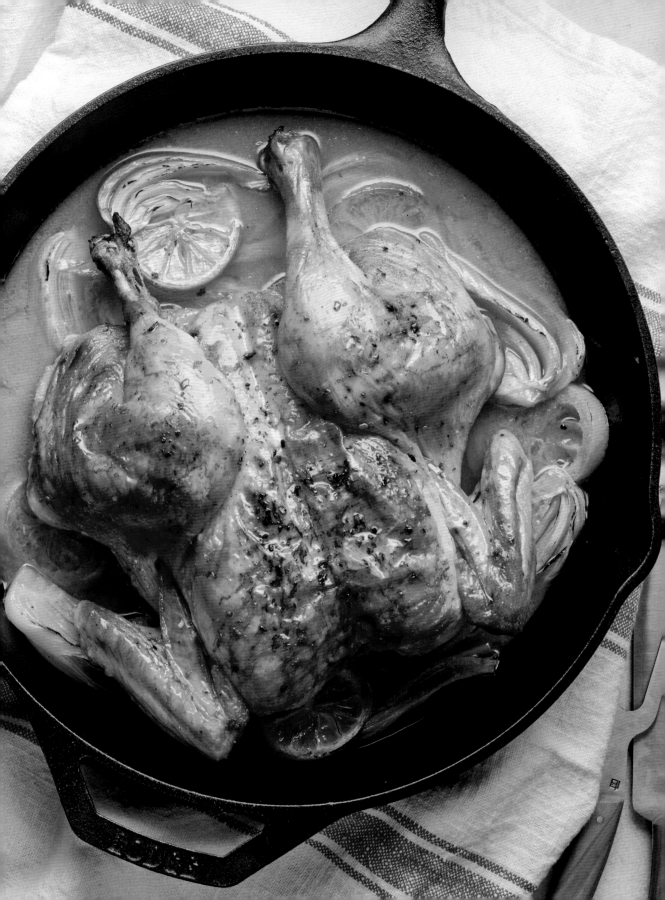

Five

Poultry & Meat

If there is one thing that

the difference between the way Americans and Italians eat, it is the role of meat in our diets—or more precisely the predominance of meat. Simply put, Americans just eat more of it, and I often have people tell me my meat recipes are not as substantial as what they are used to. I get it, but I've never felt comfortable doling out gigantic portions of meat, at home or at my restaurants, and lately I think more people are coming around to my way of thinking.

When I was a kid growing up in Italy, meat was often part of our meals, but it never played a starring role on our dinner table. As was typical in an Italian home, we filled our plates with vegetables and it looked generous and abundant. In part, this was because my mother grew up with parents who had become accustomed to the scarcity of meat during the war years; making a little meat go a long way was so deeply ingrained in my grandparents that it just became the norm even when times were flush. That's pretty much the case throughout most of Italy, where fish, vegetables, and grains appear in much more abundance than meat—especially red meat like beef and lamb.

I am by no means a vegetarian, and the older I get, the more I have come to acknowledge that having a little more animal protein in my diet than I had been eating previously just makes me feel better. I need the protein to keep my bones and muscles strong, and certain nutrients, like vitamin B_{12}, are found only in red meat. But while I do include a variety of meats in my diet, I don't eat a lot of them—usually only about 4 ounces per serving—and I make sure every bite carries a ton of flavor. Take my Gorgonzola-topped filet steak or the roasted pork tenderloin; I find that 4 ounces is a big enough portion to satisfy my yen for meat without weighing me down for hours afterward.

So, I am going to challenge you: Before you instantly decide that half a chicken breast or a single skewer of grilled lamb won't do for your hearty appetite, go with my portions and see if you really, truly are not satisfied. You can always have more, but you may be surprised to realize that the big flavors do the trick.

To keep it nice and easy, many of these dishes are one-pot meals with the vegetables built right in. The rest are simple enough to prepare that you will have bandwidth for a side dish and a salad for good measure, and because they won't fill you up too much, you'll have room for dessert, too (page 243).

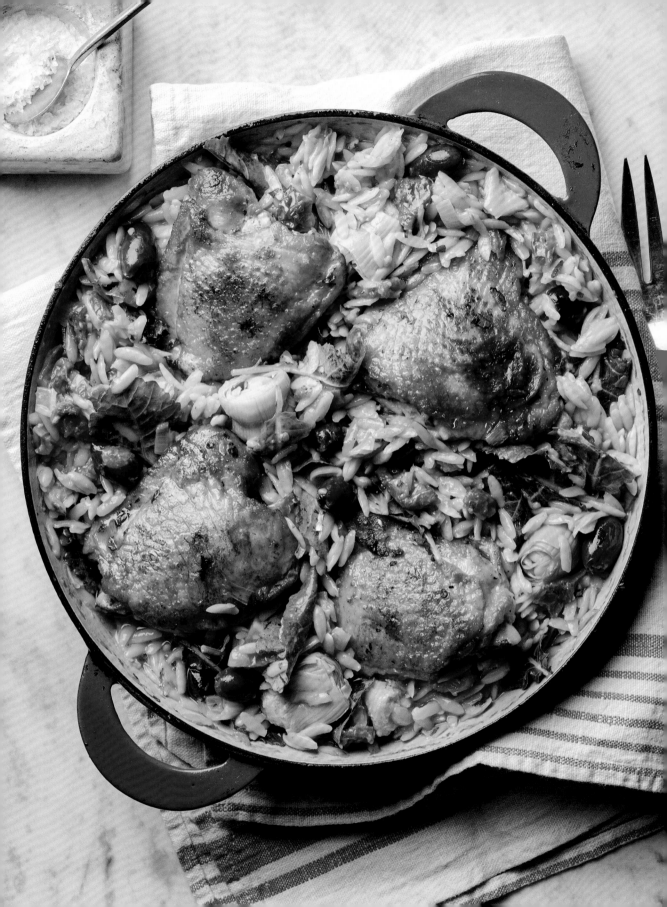

One-Pan Chicken
with **Artichokes** and **Orzo**

When I ran a version of this recipe on Giadzy, the response was through the roof, with commenters noting they especially loved the one-pot convenience of it all. I decided to revisit it, pumping up the Italian flavors even more for a dish that has a different taste in every bite. While the inspiration recipe called for boneless, skinless thighs, here I'm using whole bone-in thighs because they stay nice and moist and get that gorgeous crispy skin. If you prefer to use boneless thighs or even chicken breasts, be my guest, just take care not to overcook them.

Serves
4

- 1 tablespoon extra-virgin olive oil
- 4 meaty bone-in, skin-on chicken thighs
- 2 teaspoons kosher salt
- 1 large shallot, chopped
- 1 cup orzo
- 1 (7-ounce) jar oil-packed sun-dried tomatoes, drained and roughly chopped
- ½ cup halved artichoke hearts (canned, jarred, or frozen)
- ½ cup pitted black olives, such as kalamata
- 1 tablespoon chopped fresh oregano
- 3 cups low-sodium chicken broth
- 3 tablespoons fresh lemon juice (1 large lemon)
- 3 cups baby spinach or baby kale

Preheat the oven to 350°F.

In a Dutch oven or ovenproof skillet, heat the oil over medium-high heat. Season the chicken thighs all over with 1 teaspoon of the salt and place skin side down in the pan. Cook until the skin is golden brown and the chicken releases easily from the pan, 5 to 7 minutes. Remove the chicken to a plate and set aside.

In the same pan, cook the shallot in the rendered fat until slightly softened, about 2 minutes. Add the orzo and cook, stirring, until the orzo is lightly toasted, about 2 minutes. Add the sun-dried tomatoes, artichokes, olives, oregano, broth, lemon juice, and the remaining 1 teaspoon salt and stir to combine. Nestle the chicken thighs, along with any juices, back into the pan skin side up so they are about half submerged.

Transfer the pan to the oven and bake uncovered until the orzo is tender and the chicken is cooked through, about 20 minutes. Turn off the oven.

Stir the spinach into the hot pasta and return the pan to the still-warm oven, uncovered, until the greens have wilted, 3 or 4 minutes. Serve directly from the pan.

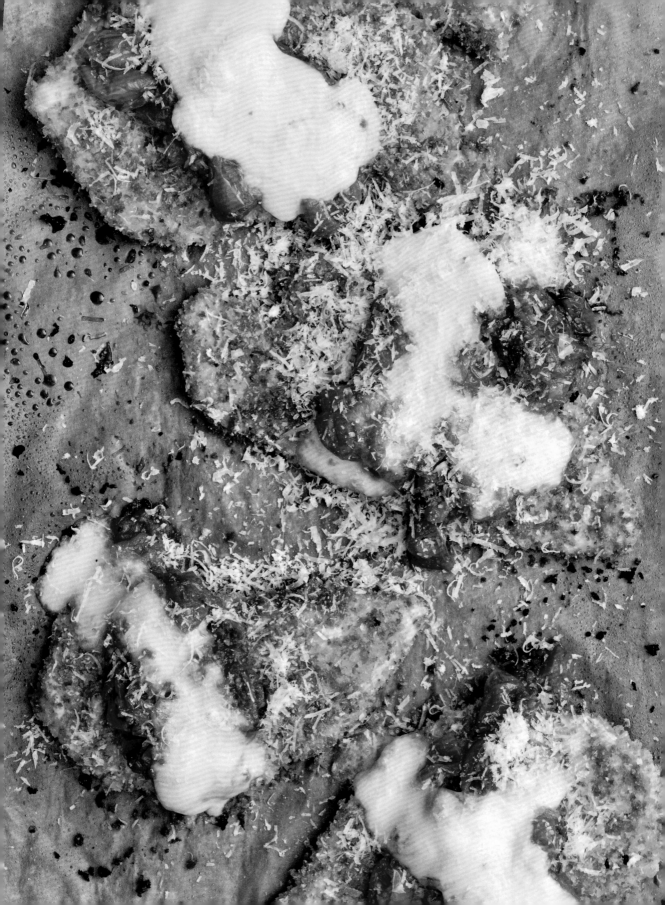

Sheet Pan Chicken "Parm"

WITH FRESH TOMATO SAUCE

Before you dismiss this lighter, brighter, bolder version of the classic—Is that all the cheese you're using!? It's not even fried!!—give it a try. I think you'll agree that you get all the flavors you crave with a lot less fat (and greasy cleanup) than is usually part of the deal. If you want to make a dish that skews a little more traditional, use one of the tomato sauces on pages 61 or 63 or your favorite store-bought marinara and sub Parmigiano-Reggiano for the pecorino. You'll still be way ahead of the game, healthwise.

Serves
4

2 tablespoons extra-virgin olive oil

2 shallots, thinly sliced

2 pints cherry tomatoes, halved, or 8 Campari tomatoes, diced

2½ teaspoons kosher salt

¼ cup shredded fresh basil leaves

2 large boneless, skinless chicken breasts (about 10 ounces each)

2 large eggs

1 cup Garlicky Bread Crumbs (page 47)

⅔ cup freshly grated pecorino cheese, plus more for serving

4 ounces fresh mozzarella cheese, cut into 4 slices

Preheat the oven to 450°F. Line a sheet pan with parchment paper.

In a saucepan, heat the oil over medium heat. Add the shallots and stir until starting to soften, about 3 minutes. Stir in the tomatoes, reduce the heat to low, cover, and cook until the tomatoes are softened, about 5 minutes. Season with ½ teaspoon of the salt and the basil and remove from the heat.

Meanwhile, one at a time, place the chicken breasts on a cutting board and holding a sharp knife parallel to the board, slice horizontally into two equal cutlets. Using the heel of your hand (or the bottom of a wine bottle), pound the cutlets to a thin, even thickness. Repeat with the second breast.

Break the eggs into a shallow bowl and beat until homogenous. Combine the bread crumbs and ¾ cup of the pecorino in a second shallow bowl.

Season the chicken cutlets with the remaining 2 teaspoons salt. One at a time, dip the cutlets first in the beaten egg and then in the cheesy crumbs, pressing the crumbs firmly to coat both sides. Place on the lined pan.

Bake the cutlets until golden, about 12 minutes. Flip and continue to bake until cooked through, another 6 minutes.

Remove the pan from the oven (leaving the oven on) and top each breast with some of the tomato sauce. Tear each slice of mozzarella in 2 pieces and arrange on top of the sauce. Return to the oven until the sauce is bubbling and the cheese is melted. Sprinkle each cutlet with a bit more pecorino and serve hot.

Southern Italian Herbed Roast Chicken

There is something about the combination of lemon and chicken that just delights me, and this is one of the best ways I know to showcase those flavors. I didn't grow up eating roast chicken; I fell in love with it when I moved to Paris to attend cooking school. There it seemed like just about every small bistro served a perfectly roasted bird, usually small poussins or even squab, crisp, juicy, and perfectly tender, in a puddle of its own juices—divine! And now that spatchcocked chickens are available in so many markets (see Hint), I can do all that in about half the time. Serving it with a fresh, herby green sauce takes this in a more Italian direction, but the aroma still brings me right back to my days at Le Cordon Bleu.

Serves

4

2 tablespoons extra-virgin olive oil

1 large fennel bulb (stalks removed and a few leafy fronds reserved for garnish), cut into 10 to 12 wedges

1 large lemon, thinly sliced

1 whole chicken (3 to 4 pounds), spatchcocked (see Hint)

2 teaspoons GDL Seasoned Salt (page 48)

1½ cups low-sodium chicken broth

1 cup Kale Salsa Verde (page 54)

Preheat the oven to 425°F.

Spread 1 tablespoon oil in a large-cast iron skillet. Arrange the fennel wedges in the pan and tuck the lemon slices among them. Drizzle with the remaining 1 tablespoon oil. Season the chicken all over with the seasoned salt and set it on top of the fennel skin side up.

Roast for 25 minutes, then add the broth to the skillet. Return to the oven and roast until the chicken is golden brown and an instant-read thermometer in the thickest part of the thigh registers 165°F, another 20 to 25 minutes. If the skin isn't browned enough, place the chicken under the broiler for 3 or 4 minutes. Let the chicken rest, loosely covered, for 10 minutes before cutting into pieces and serving with the fennel, the pan juices, and the salsa verde.

HINT HINT ◆ "Spatchcocking" is just a chef-y term for splitting and flattening any bird so that it cooks more quickly and evenly. I am seeing them in more and more markets these days and if you are handy with a pair of kitchen shears (or have an accommodating butcher), it is no big deal to split a regular whole bird. Just ask to have the backbone cut out or do it yourself, then press down on the breast with the heel of your hand to break the breastbone so the bird lies flat. And if none of the above work for you, using "split broilers," or chicken halves, will accomplish the same result. Bonus: Spatchcocked chickens are also a whole lot easier to carve than a whole roasted bird.

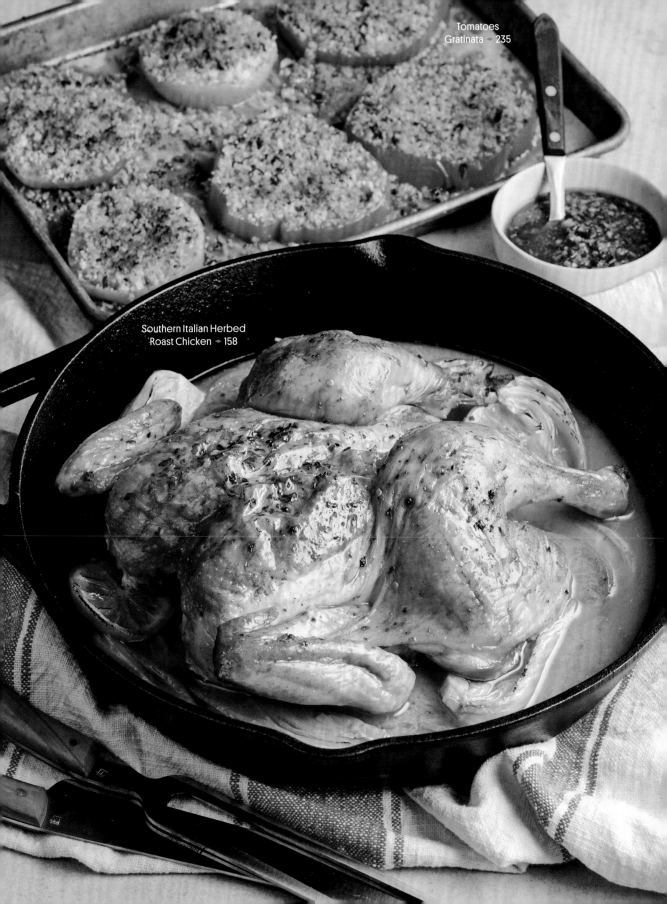

Tomatoes
Gratinata → 235

Southern Italian Herbed
Roast Chicken → 158

Chicken Piccata Meatballs

If only all mash-ups were as instantly appealing as these tender little pillows, one of the most popular entrées on the menu at my Vegas restaurant. I start with something that is universally beloved—meatballs—and then bathe them in the piquant flavors of an Italian American classic, using capers, lemon, and a bit of cheese for a lovely, silky sauce. A quick trip under the broiler gives the meatballs a golden exterior without drying them out, no mean feat when you are working with a meat as lean as ground chicken. The recipe makes a generous amount of sauce and I like to serve it and the meatballs ladled over a bed of arugula with a hunk of good bread for sopping. They would be equally tasty served over pasta or rice if that's how you roll.

Makes
20 MEATBALLS
(SERVES 4)

◆

FOR THE MEATBALLS

1 to 2 slices soft white bread, crusts removed, torn in small pieces [½ cup]

2 tablespoons whole milk

½ cup freshly grated Parmigiano-Reggiano cheese

1 large egg

1 shallot, finely chopped

2 tablespoons drained capers, chopped

Grated zest of 1 lemon

½ teaspoon kosher salt

2 tablespoons chopped fresh flat-leaf Italian parsley

1 pound ground chicken

Position a rack in the upper third of the oven and preheat the broiler. Line a sheet pan with parchment paper and set aside.

Make the meatballs: In a medium bowl, combine the bread, milk, Parmigiano, and egg, stirring with a fork to mix thoroughly. Set aside for 5 minutes to allow the bread to absorb the liquid.

Add the shallot, capers, lemon zest, salt, and parsley and mix well with a rubber spatula until the mixture is smooth and homogenous. Add the chicken, breaking it into chunks, then use your fingertips to gently combine the chicken with the bread mixture just until blended. With dampened hands, form the mixture into balls, using about 1½ tablespoons of the mixture for each, and arrange them on the oiled sheet pan.

Broil the meatballs until the tops are golden brown, about 7 minutes.

CONTINUES

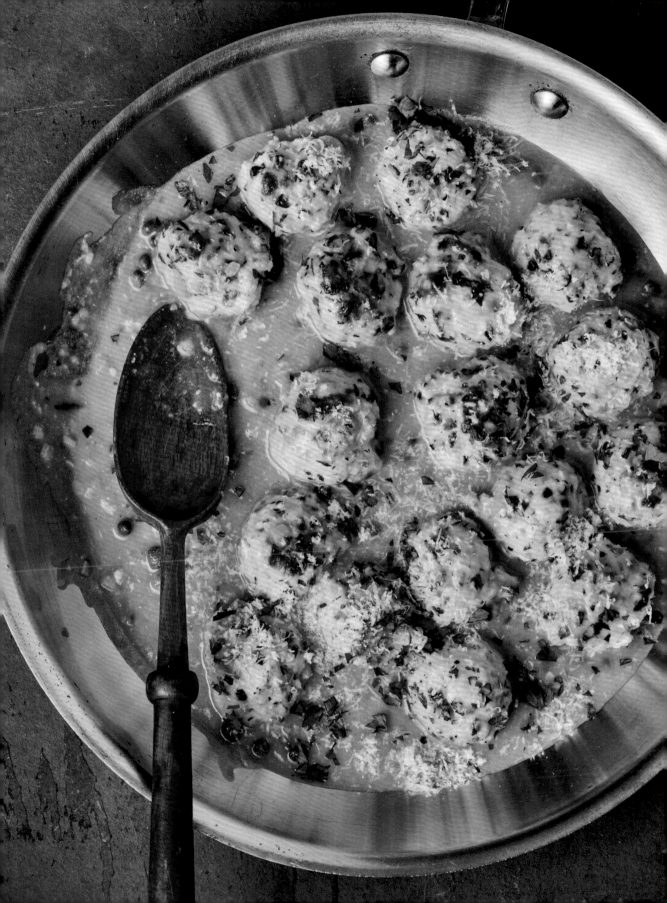

FOR THE SAUCE

2 tablespoons extra-virgin olive oil

1 shallot, finely chopped

½ teaspoon kosher salt

1 tablespoon all-purpose flour

1½ cups Parmesan Chicken Broth
(page 64) or low-sodium
store-bought chicken broth

2 tablespoons fresh lemon juice

1½ tablespoons drained capers

2 tablespoons chopped fresh
flat-leaf Italian parsley

Freshly grated Parmigiano-Reggiano
cheese, for serving

Make the sauce: In a deep skillet, heat the oil over medium heat. Add the shallot and salt and cook, stirring often, for 1 minute. Sprinkle in the flour and whisk until smooth. Continuing to whisk, add the chicken broth and lemon juice and stir until smooth. When the sauce begins to bubble, reduce the heat to low, add the capers, and simmer the sauce for 5 minutes.

Add the meatballs to the pan, cover, and cook for another 5 minutes. Stir in the parsley. Serve with a little freshly grated Parmigiano.

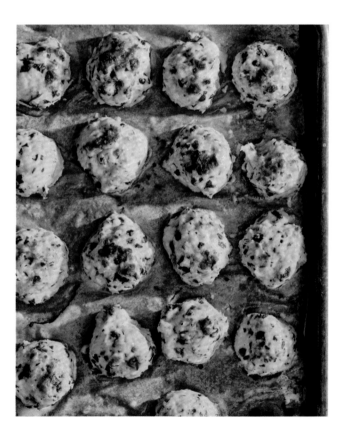

Umbrian Chicken Stew

WITH GREEN OLIVES

You'll find stews of all kinds in the central regions of Italy. I gravitate to those made with chicken because it becomes succulent and soft in well under an hour. This is probably more reminiscent of a coq au vin than a chicken cacciatore, but I use white wine rather than red so it's a bit less heavy. With a simmered dish like this one I like to add a fresh element at the end, like chopped arugula or parsley, and serve it drizzled with extra-virgin olive oil.

Serves

4

◆

1 tablespoon extra-virgin olive oil

½ cup diced pancetta (2 ounces)

½ red onion, diced

1 carrot, peeled and diced

1 celery stalk, diced

1½ teaspoons kosher salt

1½ pounds boneless, skinless chicken thighs (about 4 large)

2½ tablespoons all-purpose flour

2 medium Yukon Gold potatoes (about 12 ounces total), cut into chunks

½ bunch lacinato (Tuscan) kale, stripped off the center ribs and chopped

1 pint fresh cherry tomatoes

1 cup white wine

1 cup Parmesan Chicken Broth (page 64) or low-sodium store-bought chicken broth

1 cup Castelvetrano or Cerignola olives

4 fresh thyme sprigs or 1 teaspoon dried

2 large strips orange zest

4 slices sourdough bread, toasted, for serving

Best-quality extra-virgin olive oil, for drizzling

¼ cup chopped fresh flat-leaf Italian parsley

In a heavy-bottomed pot or Dutch oven, heat the oil over medium heat. Add the pancetta and sauté until the fat renders and the bits are browned, about 4 minutes.

Add the onion, carrot, celery, and ½ teaspoon salt and sauté until softened, about 5 minutes.

Cut each chicken thigh into 2 or 3 pieces. (See Hint.) Push the veggies to the side of the pan and add the chicken. Sprinkle with ½ teaspoon salt and cook until lightly browned, 4 or 5 minutes. Sprinkle the flour into the pan, avoiding the chicken, and cook, stirring for a minute.

Add the potatoes, kale, tomatoes, wine, broth, olives, thyme, orange zest, and the remaining ½ teaspoon salt and stir to combine. Bring to a simmer over medium-high heat. Reduce the heat to medium-low, cover, and cook for 10 minutes. Uncover and continue to cook until the potatoes are tender when pierced with a fork and the sauce has thickened, another 5 minutes or so.

To serve, use two forks to shred the chicken. Place a slice of toast in each serving bowl, ladle the stew on top, and drizzle with the finishing oil. Sprinkle with the parsley.

HINT HINT ◆ I like this with the chicken pulled into shreds for texture similar to a ragu, so I cook the chicken in largish pieces, but if you prefer a more stew-like presentation, cut the chicken into chunks.

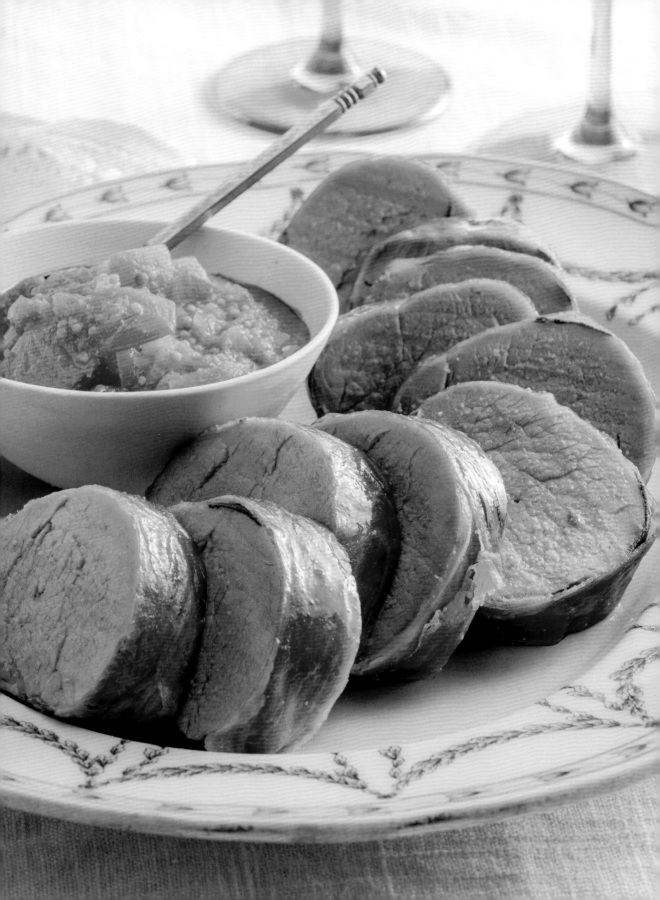

Tuscan Pork Tenderloin

WITH MOSTARDA

In America, beef is king, but Italians eat a lot more pork than beef, whether cured, smoked, or roasted. I like the tenderloin because it is less fatty and a bit more delicate than some other cuts, but it can be dry if overcooked and flavorless if not seasoned properly. Wrapping it in a flavor-enhancing barrier of prosciutto and fresh sage avoids both pitfalls beautifully and also makes a quick, easy dish for entertaining. If you like, you can make a fast sauce with the pan juices, but for me, a bit of fruity mostarda is all the embellishment this needs. Its spicy, sweet flavor really complements pork.

Serves

4 TO 6

2 medium pork tenderloins (about 1 pound each; see Hint)

2 teaspoons kosher salt

10 to 12 slices prosciutto

12 large fresh sage leaves

2 tablespoons extra-virgin olive oil

1 cup Summer Mostarda (page 56)

HINT HINT ◆ In most markets tenderloins come two to a package and they are not always identical (or even similar) in weight. If this is the case with yours, you may need to cook the larger one 2 to 3 minutes longer than the smaller one. Let your instant-read thermometer be your guide. Even though it's unlikely anyone will be harmed by undercooked pork (and many chefs prefer it on the rare side), in my experience folks are wary of pork that is more than a teeny bit pink. Pork roasted to 135°F will rise to a safe (and visually reassuring) 140°F as it rests.

Preheat the oven to 425°F.

Pat the tenderloins dry with paper towels and use a sharp knife to remove any large bits of fat or silver skin (the thin layer of connective tissue that may be visible on the meat's surface). Season well on all sides with the salt. If one end of the tenderloin is much thinner than the other, fold the tapered end underneath to make a piece with consistent thickness. This will ensure that it cooks evenly.

On a work surface, place half the prosciutto slices side by side, overlapping slightly, to make a sheet of prosciutto as wide as the tenderloin is long. Arrange half the sage leaves randomly on top of the prosciutto. Place one of the tenderloins perpendicular to the far end of the strips and roll it away from you, encasing it in the prosciutto as you roll and pressing it onto the meat. (Don't worry if the prosciutto doesn't quite wrap all the way around.) Repeat with the remaining prosciutto, sage, and tenderloin.

In a large ovenproof skillet, heat the oil over medium-high heat. When the oil is hot, add the tenderloins, seam side down, and sear until the prosciutto is browned and crisp. Turn and continue to sear until all sides are golden, about 8 minutes total.

Transfer the skillet to the oven and roast until an instant-read thermometer registers about 135°F, 15 to 18 minutes. Transfer the pork to a serving platter to rest for 10 minutes.

Slice the pork into ½-inch slices, drizzle with any juices that have accumulated on the cutting board or platter, and serve with the mostarda.

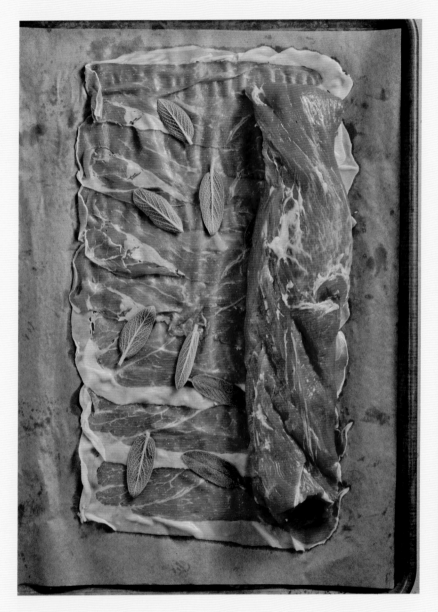
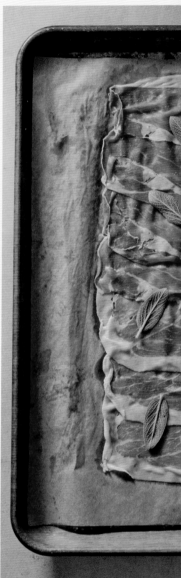

TUSCAN PORK TENDERLOIN ◆ PAGE 165

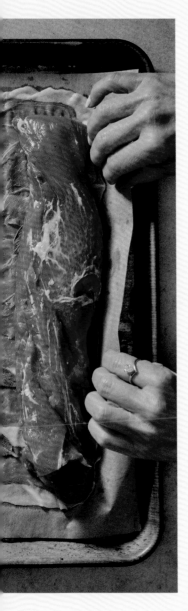
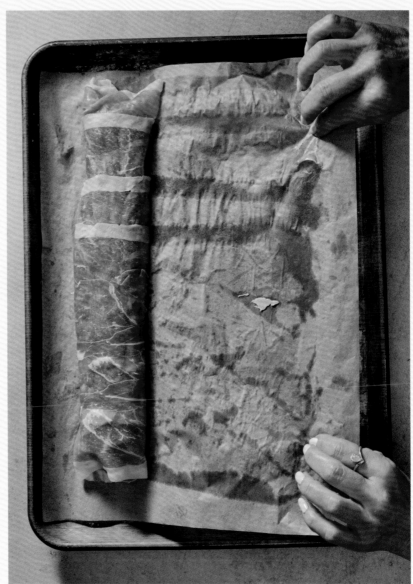

Pork Scarpariello

I often bring a touch of California to traditional Italian dishes, but in this case, I've done the reverse, bringing a classic Italian sensibility to an Italian American creation. I've substituted pork for the usual chicken because, believe it or not, chicken is not served nearly as often in Italian homes as are pork, lamb, and veal. I've also used bright yellow pepperoncini rather than cherry peppers because I love their tangy brine and sharp bite. Don't overcook the meat—when it is pounded out this thin it really will be cooked through in about 4 minutes. Any longer and it will be as tough as the sole of your shoe.

Serves

4

◆

4 thin-cut boneless pork chops (about 3 ounces each)

Generous 1 tablespoon GDL Seasoned Salt (page 48)

¼ cup all-purpose flour

1 tablespoon extra-virgin olive oil

2 tablespoons unsalted butter

2 garlic cloves, smashed and peeled

1 cup white wine

1 cup low-sodium chicken broth

6 brine-packed pepperoncini, thinly sliced crosswise

1 tablespoon brine from the pepperoncini jar, or more to taste

3 tablespoons fresh lemon juice (one large lemon)

½ pint cherry tomatoes, halved

½ teaspoon kosher salt

Cooked fregola or other small pasta shape, for serving

Place the pork between two sheets of parchment and pound to about ¼ inch thick. Season generously on both sides with the seasoned salt, then dust liberally on both sides with the flour, shaking off the excess.

In a large skillet (if your cutlets are very large you may need to do this in two batches), heat the oil and butter over medium-high heat. When the butter has melted, add the garlic and stir for 1 to 2 minutes to infuse the butter and oil; discard the garlic.

Add the pork and cook over medium-high heat just until starting to turn golden, 2 to 3 minutes. Flip the cutlets and cook until the second side is golden, another 1 to 2 minutes. Transfer the pork to a plate.

Add the wine to the pan and stir over medium heat, scraping up the browned bits from the bottom of the pan. Cook until somewhat reduced, 3 or 4 minutes. Add the chicken broth, pepperoncini, pepper brine (use more if you like it really spicy), lemon juice, tomatoes, and kosher salt. Cook at a rapid simmer until the tomatoes have softened, about 10 minutes.

Return the pork and any juices that have accumulated on the plate to the skillet and turn to coat the cutlets with the sauce. Cook for about 2 minutes to warm the pork through and to thicken the sauce a bit.

Serve the pork over the pasta, topped with the pepperoncini, tomatoes, and a liberal spoonful of sauce.

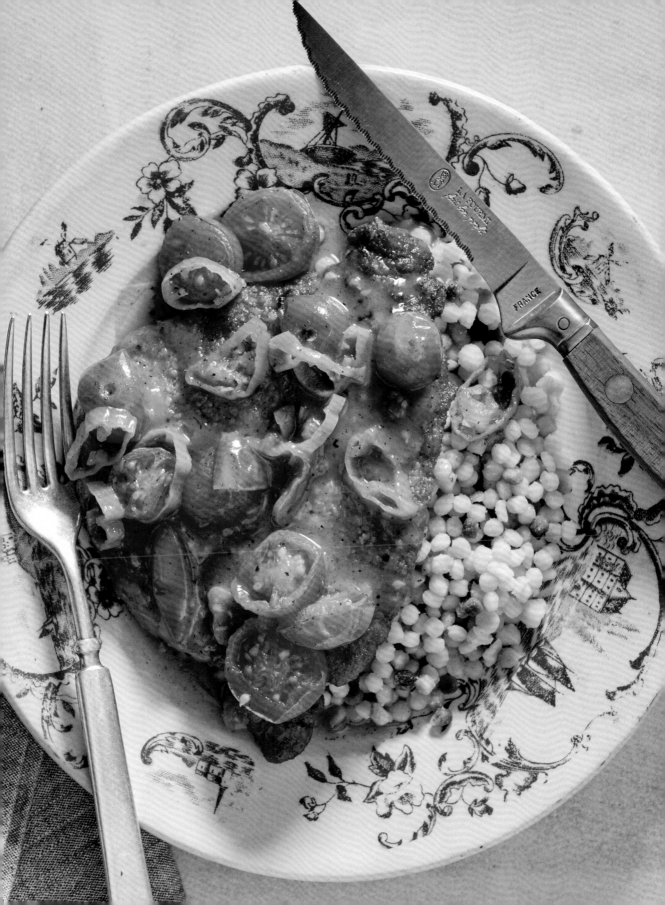

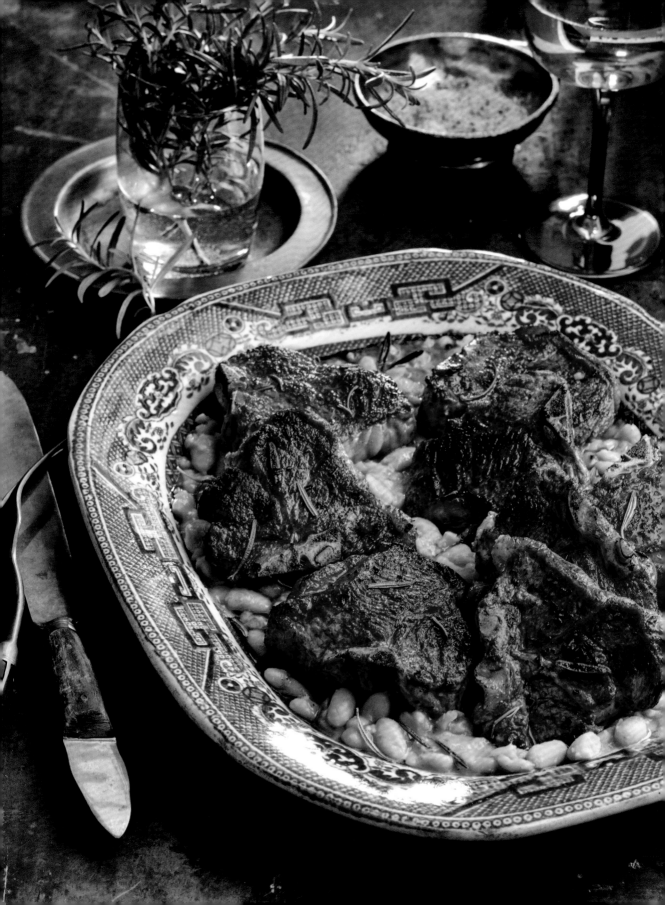

Rosemary Lamb Chops
WITH Creamy Beans

An easy weeknight meal that is more than special enough to serve to company is always going to get top marks in my book, and this one is a perfect example. When I make Creamy Cannellini Beans, I always make a double batch so I can bust out this fancy-ish dinner in way less than a half hour. Cooking the chops in the oven takes just minutes, but even more important, it makes cooking them to the perfect medium-rare all but foolproof. I like a bitter green such as broccoli rabe, chard, or kale on the side to contrast with the unctuous beans and rich meat.

Serves

4

❧

2 fresh rosemary sprigs, plus more for garnish

8 lamb loin chops (¾ to 1 inch thick)

Kosher salt

2 tablespoons extra-virgin olive oil

2 garlic cloves, smashed and peeled

1 cup Parmesan Chicken Broth (page 64), low-sodium store-bought chicken broth, or red wine

2 tablespoons fresh lemon juice

2 cups Creamy Cannellini Beans (page 239)

Preheat the oven to 400°F.

Strip the leaves from one of the rosemary sprigs and chop finely. Sprinkle the chops on both sides with salt and the chopped rosemary.

In a large ovenproof skillet, heat the oil over medium-high heat. Add the chops and cook until well seared on the bottom, 3 to 4 minutes.

Turn the chops, transfer the skillet to the oven, and roast until the chops register 145°F for medium-rare (they should feel resistant but not firm when pressed with a finger), 6 to 7 minutes. Transfer the chops to a plate to rest while you make the pan sauce.

Add the garlic and the remaining rosemary sprig to the skillet and sauté over medium heat for a minute or two to release their fragrance. Add the broth and lemon juice to the pan and deglaze, scraping up the browned bits from the bottom of the pan, and cook for a minute or two to reduce slightly. Stir in any meat juices that have accumulated around the chops. Discard the herb sprig and garlic cloves.

Meanwhile, in a nonstick skillet, reheat the beans, adding a bit of water or broth if too thick.

Spoon the beans on four serving plates and top each with 2 chops. Drizzle with the pan sauce, sprinkle with rosemary, and serve.

Grilled Lamb Spiedini

WITH CREAMY PISTACHIO SAUCE

I've always found lamb to be a "less is more" kind of meat that doesn't need much to bring out its rich, distinctive flavor. Because it cooks quickly and just feels a little more special than beef or pork, it's often my choice for entertaining. These are easy to make with a stovetop grill pan any time of the year, but if you are grilling outdoors they make a nice alternative to the typical ribs and burgers. The sauce started its life as a mint and pistachio pesto that helps cut the richness of the meat.

Serves
4 TO 6

FOR THE LAMB

1½ pounds boneless leg of lamb, cut into 1½-inch cubes

2 tablespoons extra-virgin olive oil

1 tablespoon balsamic vinegar

2 teaspoons light brown sugar

2 small garlic cloves, grated

2 fresh rosemary sprigs, crushed in your palms

FOR THE SAUCE

½ cup chopped fresh flat-leaf Italian parsley

¼ cup chopped fresh mint

¼ cup chopped salted roasted pistachios

2 tablespoons drained capers

1 garlic clove, roughly chopped

Grated zest and juice of 1 large lemon

½ teaspoon kosher salt

¼ cup extra-virgin olive oil

½ cup plain Greek yogurt

1 tablespoon GDL Seasoned Salt [page 48]

Marinate the lamb: In a medium bowl, combine the lamb cubes, oil, vinegar, brown sugar, garlic, and rosemary and toss to coat the lamb well. Cover the bowl and marinate in the refrigerator for at least 1 hour and up to overnight.

Make the creamy pistachio sauce: In a food processor, combine the parsley, mint, pistachios, capers, and garlic and pulse 5 or 6 times or until coarsely chopped. Add the lemon zest and juice and kosher salt and pulse to combine. With the motor running, quickly stream in the oil to make a creamy paste. Stir ½ cup of the pesto into the yogurt (reserve the rest, if any, for another use), swirling it attractively. Refrigerate until ready to serve.

To finish: Preheat a ridged grill pan over medium-high heat until very hot, about 5 minutes.

While the pan heats, thread 4 or 5 meat cubes onto each skewer. Sprinkle the assembled skewers on all sides with the seasoned salt.

Grill the skewers until browned and nicely marked on one side, about 5 minutes. Turn the meat grilled side up and cook until well browned on the second side, another 5 to 6 minutes. At this point the lamb will be cooked to medium-rare; if you prefer it more well done, cook on the remaining sides for a minute or two each, or until browned all over.

Pile the skewers on a platter and serve with the sauce.

Beef AND Porcini Stracotto

As a kid, I didn't love pot roast. *Stracotto* means "overcooked," and sorry, Mom, that was a pretty accurate description of the one that was served in our house, stringy and kind of flavorless. I've elevated her recipe here by adding a few anchovies and smoky, earthy porcini mushrooms to give the sauce tons of depth. If you want to eat this as an Italian would, serve it over polenta (with a glass of hearty red wine) with some of the veggies pureed into the sauce to thicken it.

Serves
6 TO 8

3½-pound boneless beef chuck roast

2½ teaspoons kosher salt, plus more to taste

2 tablespoons extra-virgin olive oil

1 onion, finely chopped

1 celery stalk, finely chopped

2 carrots, peeled and cut into ¼-inch half-moons

4 garlic cloves, roughly chopped

2 tablespoons tomato paste

2 cups dry red wine

2 cups or more low-sodium beef broth

½ ounce dried porcini mushrooms

3 to 4 anchovy fillets, chopped

1 cup quartered cremini mushrooms

2 fresh rosemary sprigs

6 fresh thyme sprigs

Freshly ground black pepper

Polenta with Braised Mushrooms, (page 211), mashed potatoes, or grilled bread, for serving

3 tablespoons chopped fresh flat-leaf Italian parsley

Preheat the oven to 325°F.

Pat the beef dry with paper towels and season with 2 teaspoons of the salt. In a Dutch oven, heat the oil over medium-high heat. Add the beef and cook until browned on all sides, about 8 minutes. Remove the beef to a plate.

Reduce the heat to medium. Add the onion, celery, and carrots and season with the remaining ½ teaspoon salt. Cook, stirring frequently, until tender, about 8 minutes. Add the garlic and cook until aromatic, about 1 minute. Add the tomato paste and stir for a minute to coat the vegetables. Then add the wine, broth, and dried mushrooms, using a wooden spoon to stir up any browned bits from the bottom of the pan. Return the beef to the pot along with any juices on the plate and bring the liquid to a strong simmer. Cover the pot and place in the oven.

Cook for 1½ hours. Turn the meat over, add the anchovies, fresh mushrooms, rosemary, and thyme. If the meat is not about two-thirds covered with liquid, add a little more broth or some water. Re-cover the pot, return it to the oven, and cook until the meat is fork-tender, another 1 to 1½ hours.

Transfer the meat to a plate and set aside. Use a large spoon to skim off some fat from the braising liquid and discard the herb sprigs. If desired, use an immersion blender to puree some of the vegetables into the braising liquid. Season with salt and pepper to taste.

To serve, spread the polenta on a large, deep platter. Slice or shred the meat and arrange on top. Ladle the braising liquid and mushrooms over the meat and sprinkle with parsley.

Filet Mignon
WITH **Gorgonzola** AND **Balsamic**

If you are looking to wow someone, this "sneaky fancy" dish is a no-brainer: It tastes as impressive as it looks but is actually incredibly easy to make. It's also a perfect demonstration of how a little bit of fat—in this case decadent Gorgonzola dolce—can bring a whole lot of flavor to a lean meat. The dish reminds me of Modena, the home of balsamic vinegar, where the vinegar is used in so many dishes. You don't need a fine aged balsamic for this because it will be reduced. Save the good stuff for the Balsamic Chocolate Truffles [page 251], which would make an equally luxurious finishing touch for this meal.

Serves

6

1½ cups balsamic vinegar

3 tablespoons sugar

2 tablespoons unsalted butter

1 tablespoon extra-virgin olive oil

4 filets mignons, 1 inch thick
(about 4 ounces each)

Kosher salt and freshly ground
black pepper

2 ounces Gorgonzola dolce
or blue cheese

In a small heavy saucepan, bring the balsamic vinegar and sugar to a boil over medium-high heat. Cook the mixture at a low boil, stirring occasionally, until it is thick and syrupy, about 18 minutes.

Preheat the broiler.

In a heavy broilerproof skillet, melt the butter with the oil over medium-high heat. Season the steaks all over with salt and pepper. Cook the steaks for 4 minutes, then turn and cook an additional 2 or 3 minutes (an instant-read thermometer should register 130°F for medium-rare and 135°F for medium).

Dot the cheese over the steaks and place the pan under the broiler just until the cheese melts, about 1 minute.

Let the steaks rest for 5 minutes before transferring to serving plates and drizzling some of the balsamic reduction around each one.

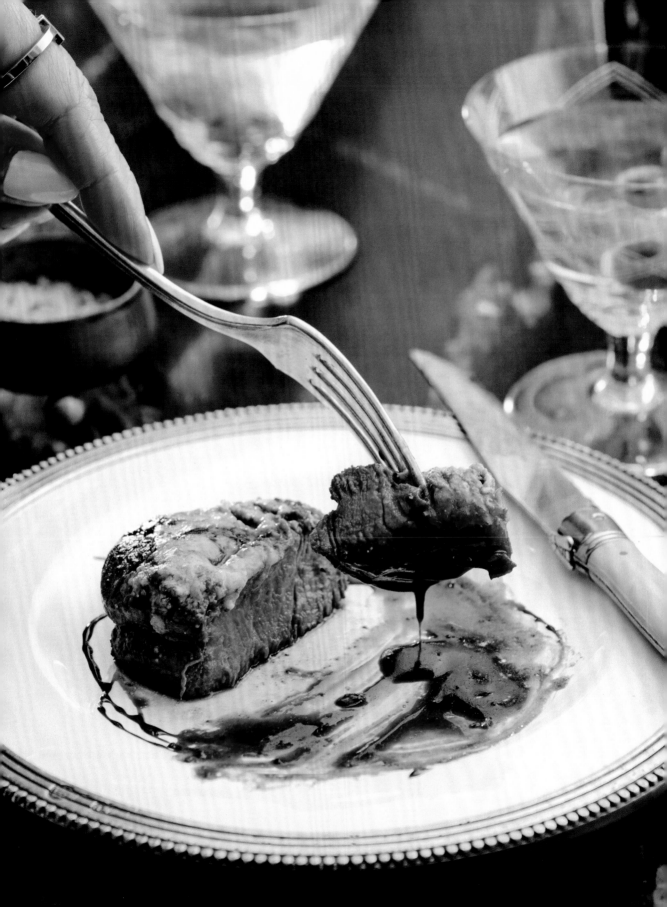

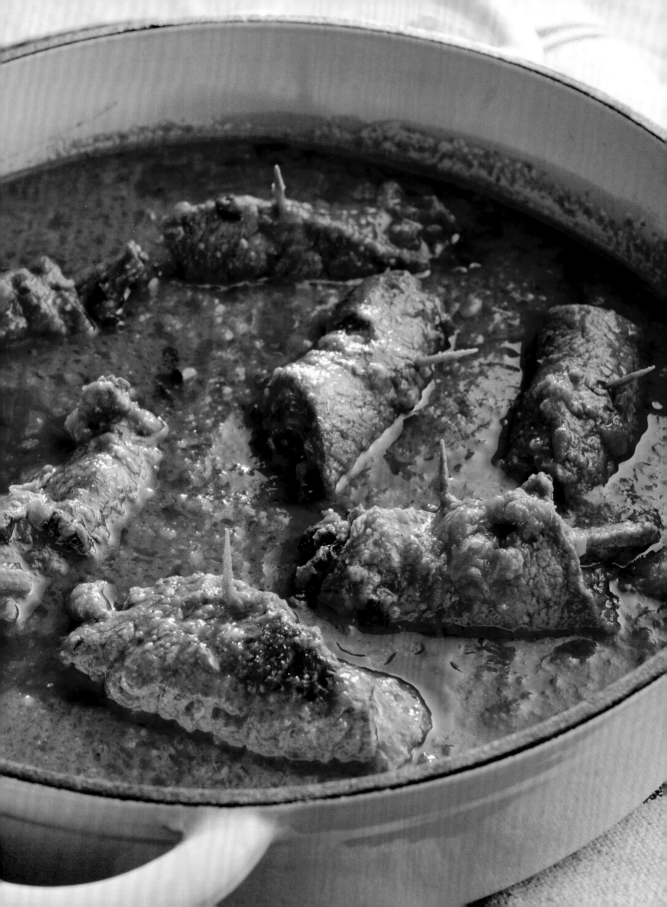

Steak Involtini WITH CHARD

Involtini means "rolled and stuffed," and beef prepared this way is a holiday tradition for many Italian families. Be sure to buy specially thin-cut meat marked "beef for braciole"; if you use another cut it may come out too tough. I usually cook this in my Simple Tomato Sauce, but since the stuffing is a bit involved, if you want to take a shortcut and substitute a purchased marinara, I'll look the other way.

Serves

4

◆

8 Swiss chard leaves

2 tablespoons extra-virgin olive oil

½ small onion, finely chopped

1½ teaspoons kosher salt

½ cup Garlicky Bread Crumbs (page 47)

½ cup freshly grated pecorino cheese

8 thin-cut slices beef top round for braciole

6-ounce chunk provolone (see Hint)

3 cups (24 ounces) Simple Tomato Sauce (page 63) or purchased marinara sauce

Pull the stems and center ribs out of the chard leaves. Chop the leaves and stems and keep them separated. In a medium skillet, heat the oil over medium-high heat until shimmering. Add the chopped chard stems and onion and cook, stirring often, until softened but not browned, about 5 minutes. Season with ½ teaspoon of the salt and stir in the chopped chard leaves. Continue to cook until the greens are soft, about 4 minutes. Remove from the heat.

Add the bread crumbs and pecorino to the skillet and mix until well combined.

Arrange the beef slices on a cutting board and sprinkle with the remaining 1 teaspoon salt. Cut the provolone into 8 long "fingers" a bit shorter than the width of the beef slices. Place about 3 tablespoons of the chard mixture on each piece of meat, spreading it over the entire slice. Top with a piece of provolone. Starting at a short end, roll the slices into cigar-shaped cylinders. Use a toothpick to secure the rolls.

Pour the marinara into a large saucepan and carefully add the beef rolls. Add a bit of water if needed to completely submerge the rolls. Bring to a gentle simmer and cook, partially covered, until the meat is tender, about 1 hour 20 minutes. Transfer the rolls to a plate.

Spoon some of the sauce onto each serving plate. Slice the rolls crosswise into 4 or 5 pieces and arrange atop the sauce. Serve hot, passing additional sauce at the table.

HINT HINT ◆ If you can't buy provolone in a chunk, stack several deli slices and cut crosswise into thick strips. Use 2 of the shorter, rounded end pieces in a single roll.

Beef Ricotta Meatballs

I've fiddled with this recipe for years, but when I was served meatballs made with a touch of ricotta on a trip to Florence, I realized that was what had been missing all along and now I never make them any other way. Fortunately, ricotta is something I always have in the fridge because I find even a smallish amount, like the half cup used here, adds a creamy, delicate texture to a lot of dishes. Letting the mixture chill overnight develops even deeper flavor. A word of warning: These are not the fist-size, bready meatballs you may have grown up on. I like meatballs to be soft and tender and small enough to eat in two or three bites, like the ones *I* grew up on. And don't let any extra sauce go to waste, because it will be fortified with all that good, beefy flavor. Save it to serve with pasta or make a quick dinner of eggs poached in the flavorful sauce.

Makes
ABOUT 24 MEATBALLS
(SERVES 4 OR 5)

FOR THE MEATBALLS

⅓ cup panko bread crumbs

3 tablespoons whole milk

1 extra-large egg

½ cup whole-milk ricotta cheese

⅔ cup freshly grated
Parmigiano-Reggiano cheese

1 pound lean ground beef

1 teaspoon kosher salt

3 cups Simple Tomato Sauce
(page 63)

FOR THE SALAD

1 (5-ounce) package baby arugula
(about 6 cups)

4 teaspoons fresh lemon juice

2 tablespoons extra-virgin olive oil

½ cup shaved Parmigiano-Reggiano
cheese

Make the meatballs: In a medium bowl, combine the panko, milk, egg, ricotta, and Parmigiano. Stir well to combine and set aside for 10 minutes to allow the bread crumbs to absorb the liquid. Add the beef and salt. Use your hands to combine the ingredients gently but thoroughly. Cover the bowl and refrigerate the mixture overnight.

Position a rack in the upper third of the oven and preheat the oven to 450°F. Line a sheet pan with parchment.

Form heaping tablespoons of the beef mixture into balls and arrange them on the sheet pan about 1 inch apart. Roast the meatballs until firm, about 20 minutes.

Transfer the meatballs to a Dutch oven or deep skillet and add the tomato sauce. Bring the sauce to a simmer, stirring gently to coat the meatballs in the sauce, then cover the pan and cook over low heat for 15 minutes. Remove from the heat.

Meanwhile, make the salad: In a medium bowl, toss together the arugula, lemon juice, oil, and Parmigiano shavings. Divide the greens among four or five shallow bowls.

Top with the meatballs and serve.

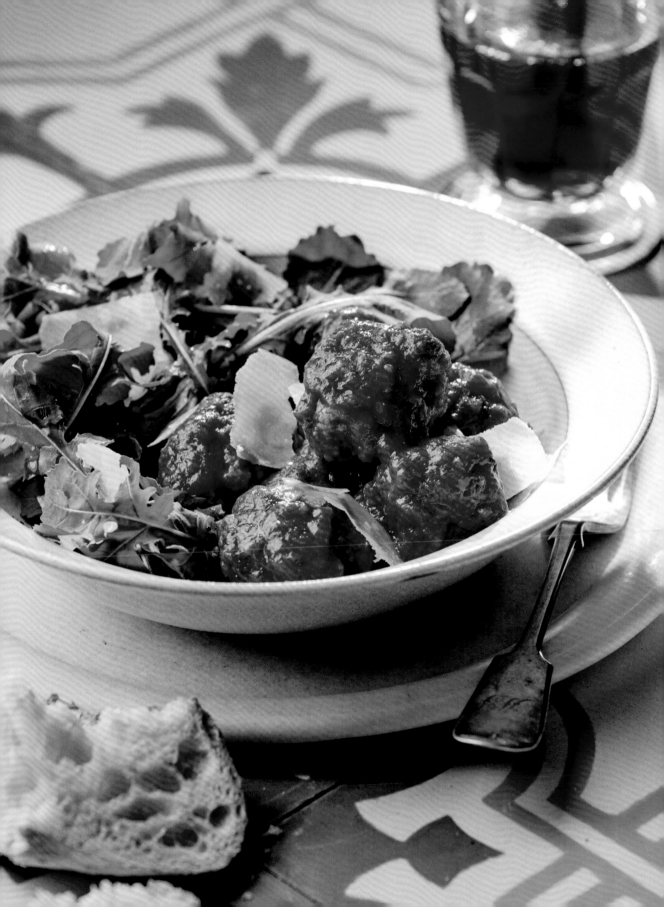

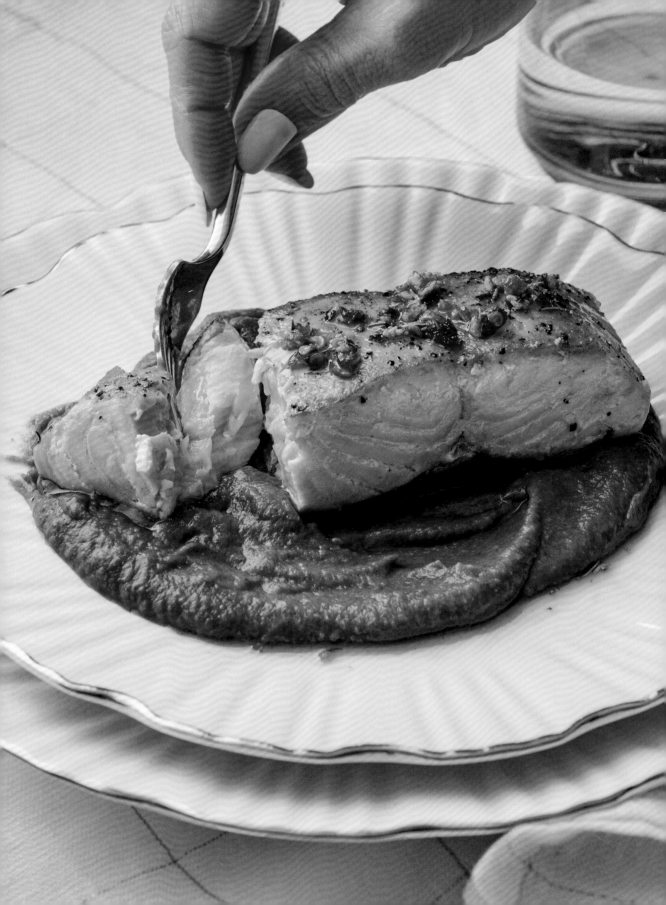

Six

Fish & Shellfish

It makes me happy to see

HOW MUCH MORE POPULAR

◆

fish has become in the last decade, although the amount of fish consumed in this country pales in comparison to how often it is eaten in many parts of Italy. There it is on the menu a lot because it's what is available locally, especially to the South and in coastal areas; the number of ways swordfish alone is prepared in Sicily literally boggled my mind!

I have a bit of a complicated relationship with fish. I love almost every kind of fish and would eat it every day if I could—in fact I very nearly did until I was diagnosed with heavy metal poisoning and had to cut way back on the amount of fish in my diet, especially those fish with long lifespans such as tuna, halibut, and salmon. Now I try to focus on smaller fish and those lower on the food chain, because spending less time in the water means they have less time to pick up contaminants from their environment. But even though bigger fish are more of a now-and-then event than they once were, I still eat some kind of fish or seafood at least twice a week, whether it's shrimp, mussels, or scallops, or a pasta with anchovies or clams.

That's because in addition to being delicious, fish and shellfish are the original fast food, requiring minimal prep and cooking up in 10 or 15 minutes. You'll find many of the recipes in this chapter make strategic use of the condiments in Chapter 1: Flavor Starts Here (page 43), so not only are the cook times streamlined, the ingredient lists are, too. And of course, every one of these recipes is a lighter, lower-fat alternative to a meal centered around red meat.

I hope you will find some of your favorite seafood represented in this chapter, as well as reasons to experiment with some you are not as familiar with, like monkfish or branzino. And remember that when it comes to cooking seafood, less is more: Keep it fresh, keep it simple, and avoid overcooking at all costs. With those three simple rules in mind, plus a handful of my trusty condiments in hand, you are well on your way to an easy breezy dinner in well under 30 minutes.

Sheet Pan Fritto Misto

WITH CAPER TARTAR SAUCE

Fritto misto literally means "mixed fry," and as the name suggests, you can use a mix of any seafood you like as long as it cooks quickly. Traditionally this would be deep-fried, but I don't enjoy dealing with a big pot of hot oil. Fortunately, shallow-frying the seafood in about ½ inch of oil gives a nice, crispy result with a much easier cleanup. Don't leave out the lemon and herbs; they give the oil a wonderful hint of flavor and are a pretty garnish, too!

Serves
4

FOR THE TARTAR SAUCE

½ cup Greek yogurt

3 tablespoons drained capers, chopped

2 teaspoons caper brine from the jar

2 pepperoncini (optional), chopped

Grated zest and juice of ½ lemon

¼ teaspoon kosher salt

½ teaspoon honey

FOR THE SEAFOOD

2 cups rice flour

1 tablespoon GDL Seasoned Salt (page 48)

16 extra-large or jumbo shrimp, peeled and deveined

½ pound cleaned calamari, tubes cut into ½-inch rings

Small red snapper fillet, cut into ½-inch strips

Olive oil, as needed

5 or 6 fresh rosemary sprigs

1 lemon, thinly sliced

Kosher salt, for sprinkling

Make the tartar sauce: In a small bowl, stir together the yogurt, capers, brine, pepperoncini (if using), lemon zest and juice, salt, and honey. Set aside.

Preheat the broiler. Place a sheet pan on the bottom rack of the oven to preheat.

Prepare the seafood: In a large bowl, stir together the flour and seasoned salt. Add the shrimp and toss to coat completely with the seasoned flour. Transfer to a large sieve or a colander and shake gently to remove some of the excess flour. Repeat with the calamari and fish pieces.

Line a sheet pan with paper towels and set near the stove. In a medium skillet, heat ½ inch of oil over medium-high heat. Add the rosemary and lemon slices and fry for 30 seconds or so to flavor the oil. Drain on the paper towels.

Increase the heat under the skillet to high and when the oil is very hot, add about half the shrimp. Shallow-fry until just golden, 30 to 45 seconds, turning once. Remove to the paper towels to drain and season with kosher salt. Repeat with the remaining shellfish and the fish, cooking them in batches and adding more oil to the skillet as needed. Depending on how thinly you cut the fish strips, they may need up to 2 minutes to take on some color.

Just before serving, carefully remove the hot sheet pan from the oven and spread the seafood on the pan in a single layer. Drizzle with a tiny bit more olive oil. Return the pan to the oven and broil until golden brown and hot, about 3 minutes.

Transfer to a platter, garnish with the fried rosemary and lemon, and serve with the tartar sauce.

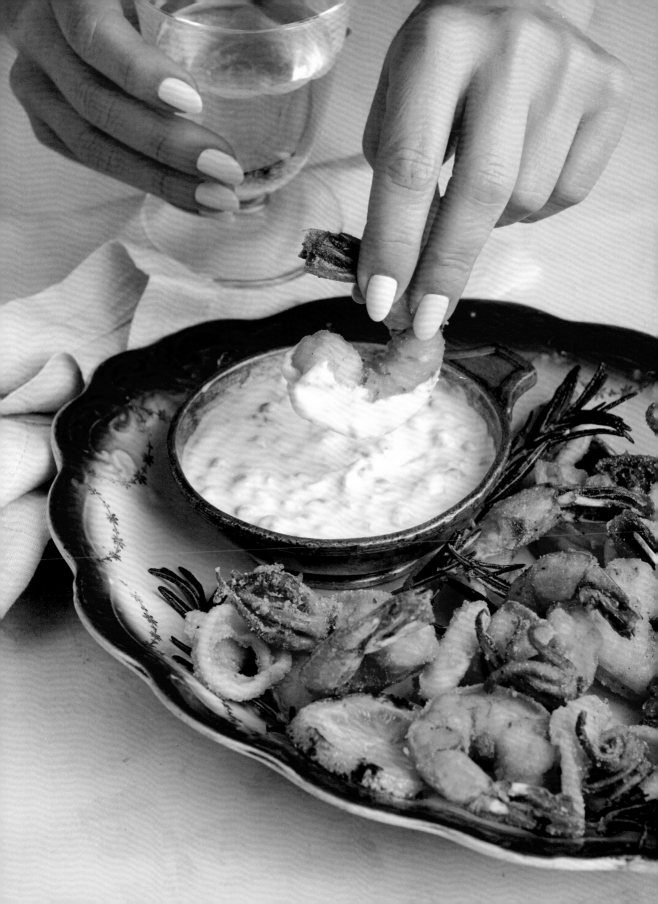

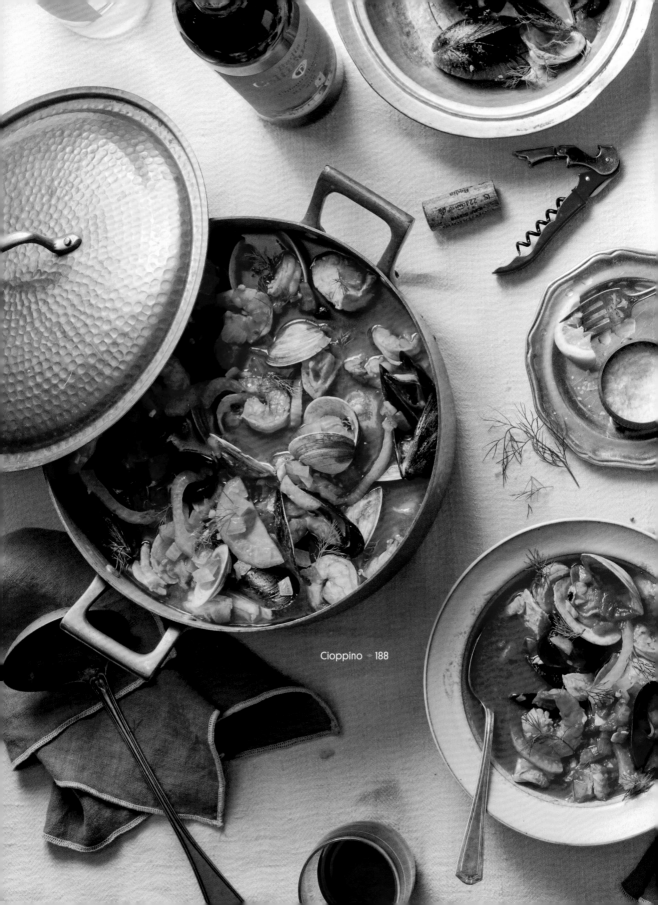

Cioppino – 188

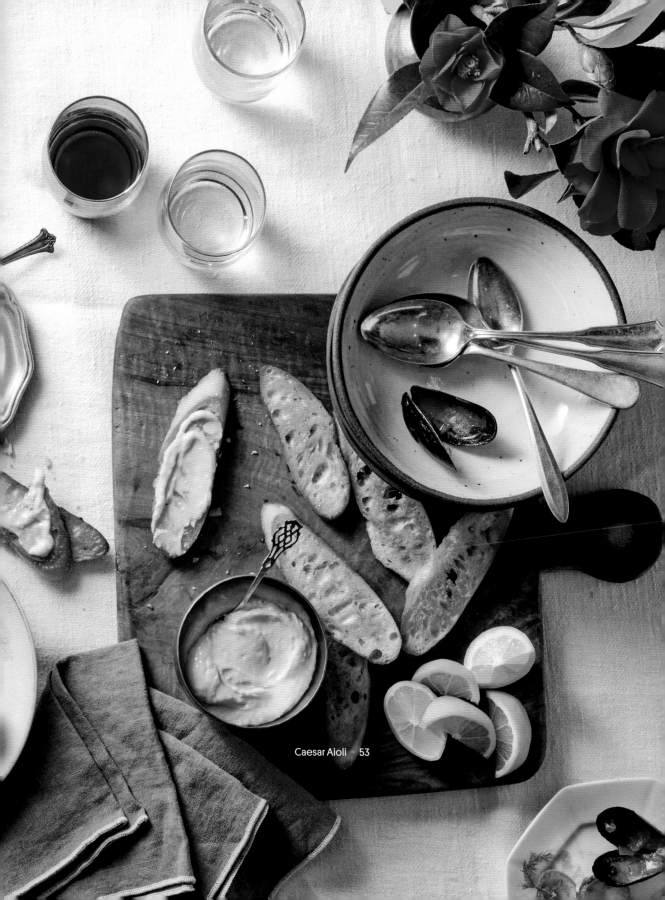

Caesar Aioli   53

Cioppino

This gorgeous stew is a good way to make less expensive seafood look special and festive and it makes a perfect party dish. I like to use monkfish here, a lovely firm fish that isn't as pricey as halibut or cod, but the choice is really yours. Some people like to include salmon, swordfish, or red snapper and they all work well. Just note that if you use a thinner fish like snapper, it should be added closer to the end so it doesn't overcook or fall apart.

Serves
6
—

3 tablespoons extra-virgin olive oil

1 large fennel bulb (stalks removed and fronds reserved for garnish), halved lengthwise and thinly sliced

1 onion, chopped

2 teaspoons kosher salt, plus more to taste

4 large garlic cloves, finely chopped

¾ teaspoon red pepper flakes, plus more to taste

3 tablespoons tomato paste

1 (28-ounce) can diced tomatoes, undrained

1½ cups dry white wine

2 (8-ounce) bottles clam juice

1 bay leaf

1 teaspoon chopped fresh oregano and/or fresh flat-leaf Italian parsley

12 littleneck clams, scrubbed

1½ pounds firm-fleshed fish fillets, such as monkfish or tilefish, cut into 2-inch chunks

1 pound mussels, scrubbed

1 pound large or extra-large shrimp, peeled and deveined

Sliced baguette, toasted, for serving

Caesar Aioli (page 53), for serving

In a Dutch oven, heat the oil over medium heat. Add the fennel, onion, and salt and sauté until the onion is translucent, about 10 minutes. Add the garlic and pepper flakes and sauté for 2 minutes longer. Stir in the tomato paste, then add the tomatoes with their juices, the wine, clam juice, bay leaf, oregano, and 3 cups water. Bring the broth to a boil over high heat, then reduce the heat to medium-low, cover the pot, and simmer for 30 minutes to blend the flavors.

Add the clams to the pot, cover, and cook for 5 minutes. Add the fish, nestling it into the liquid, re-cover the pot, and cook for 2 minutes. Add the mussels and shrimp, stir gently, re-cover, and cook just until the clams and mussels are opened and the fish and shrimp are just cooked through, about 4 minutes. (Discard any clams and mussels that do not open, as well as the bay leaf.) Season to taste with salt and pepper flakes.

Serve the stew in shallow bowls sprinkled with the reserved fennel fronds. Top each piece of toasted bread with a tablespoon of the aioli and serve with the stew, passing the remaining aioli at the table.

Grilled Swordfish
WITH Olive Bagna Cauda

Sicilians love swordfish the way Americans love salmon, and they serve it every which way: in pasta, roasted, pan-seared, and grilled. Because large fish like these can accumulate heavy metals and are less sustainable than their cousins lower down the food chain, I don't eat swordfish very often, but when I do, I like to serve it with a big-flavored accompaniment to play up its meaty flavor and texture. For this riff on bagna cauda, I have added some fresh elements to brighten the plate, in both color and taste. If possible, request fish steaks ½ inch to ¾ inch thick, or ask the fishmonger to cut a thick steak into 2 thinner ones.

Serves

4

FOR THE BAGNA CAUDA

¼ cup extra-virgin olive oil

2 anchovy fillets

3 garlic cloves, smashed and peeled

½ cup Green Olive Relish [page 55]

¼ cup red or yellow cherry tomatoes, halved

2 tablespoons chopped fresh flat-leaf Italian parsley

½ small lemon, peel and white pith removed, cut into small pieces

FOR THE FISH

4 swordfish steaks, ½ to ¾ inch thick

1 teaspoon kosher salt

¼ teaspoon freshly ground black pepper

2 teaspoons extra-virgin olive oil

Arugula, for serving

Make the bagna cauda: In a small skillet, combine the oil, anchovies, and garlic and warm over medium heat until the anchovies have melted into the oil and the sauce is gently simmering, about 5 minutes. Discard the garlic. Stir in the olive relish, tomatoes, parsley, and lemon pieces and remove from the heat.

Cook the fish: Preheat a ridged grill pan over medium-high heat.

Sprinkle the swordfish steaks on both sides with the salt and pepper and drizzle with the oil. Grill until nicely marked and opaque throughout, about 3 minutes per side, depending on the thickness of the steaks.

Arrange the arugula on a serving platter with the fish steaks on top. Spoon the bagna cauda over the fish and serve warm or at room temperature.

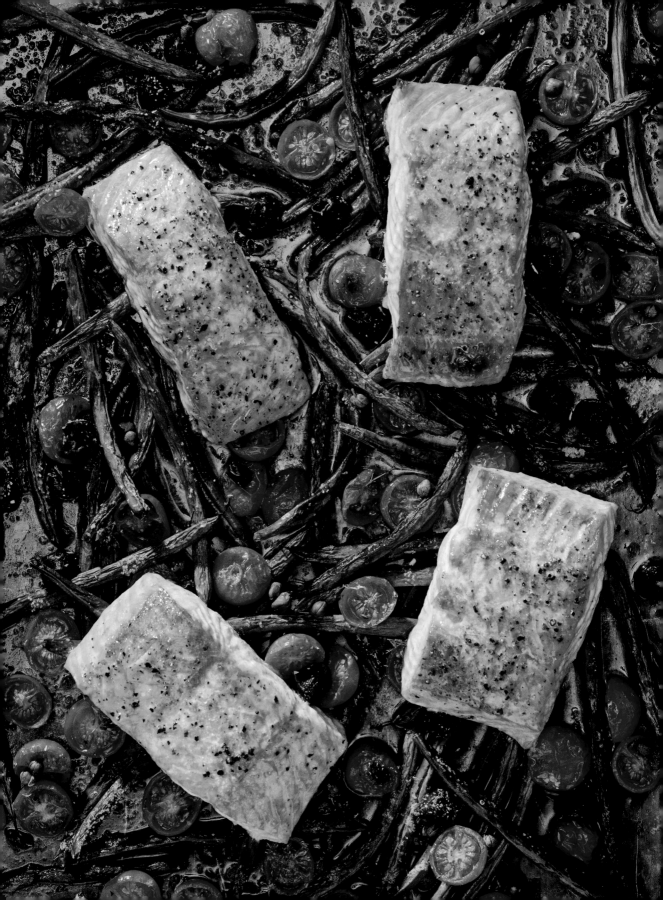

Roasted Salmon Puttanesca

One of the things that makes salmon so versatile is that it pairs as well with delicate sauces as it does with big, gutsy flavors. Here I'm taking the latter route, roasting the fish on a bed of tomatoes, olives, and capers—all the ingredients for a classic puttanesca sauce—plus green beans for crunch and color. Let the oven get good and hot before you cook the fish or it will dry out before you get a nice brown crust on top.

Serves

4

◆

1 pound green beans, trimmed

2 pints cherry tomatoes, halved, or 1 pound Campari tomatoes

¼ cup pitted kalamata olives, halved

1 tablespoon drained capers

2 tablespoons plus 2 teaspoons extra-virgin olive oil

2 teaspoons dried Sicilian oregano

1½ teaspoons kosher salt

4 skinless salmon fillets (5 to 6 ounces each)

¼ teaspoon freshly ground black pepper

½ cup Garlicky Bread Crumbs (optional; page 47)

Preheat the broiler.

Bring a large pot of salted water to a boil. Add the beans and blanch for 3 minutes, then drain well.

Spread the beans on a sheet pan. Arrange the tomatoes, olives, and capers over the beans and drizzle with 2 tablespoons of the oil. Sprinkle with the oregano and 1 teaspoon of the salt. Arrange the fish fillets on top of the vegetables. Drizzle the fish with the remaining 2 teaspoons olive oil and sprinkle with the remaining ½ teaspoon salt and the pepper.

Place the pan under the broiler and broil until the salmon has a golden brown crust, 10 to 12 minutes.

Transfer the vegetables to a platter, top with the salmon and any pan juices, and sprinkle with the bread crumbs (if using).

Simple Seared Salmon
ON Minted Pea Puree

Salmon seems to be universally popular, even with folks who are avowed fish haters, so I am always looking for new ways to serve it. I love it most when the just-cooked flesh has a good, crunchy crust, easily achieved on the stovetop in a hot skillet. That contrast of textures makes a sometimes bland fish a lot more interesting for me to eat, as does this brilliant green puree, a lighter, healthier alternative to mashed potatoes. The spicy chile oil is the crowning touch, adding a smoky note and just a bit of heat.

Serves
4

8 ounces cauliflower (about ½ small head), broken into florets

1 cup (packed) baby kale

8 ounces frozen peas

¼ cup fresh mint leaves

6 fresh chives

1½ teaspoons kosher salt

4 center-cut skin-on salmon fillets (4 to 5 ounces each)

Freshly ground black pepper

4 teaspoons Calabrian Chile Garlic Oil (page 50)

Bring a large saucepan of salted water to a boil. Add the cauliflower and cook for 4 minutes, then add the kale and peas. Cook until the cauliflower is tender when pierced with the tip of a knife, another 2 to 3 minutes.

Drain the veggies, reserving ¼ cup of the cooking liquid, and transfer them to a blender or food processor. Add the mint and chives and puree until fairly smooth, adding some of the reserved cooking water if needed to get things moving. Taste, season with up to ½ teaspoon of the salt if needed, and blend again. Keep warm while you cook the fish.

Season the salmon fillets on both sides with the remaining 1 teaspoon salt and the pepper. In a large skillet, arrange the salmon, skin side down, and place over medium-high heat. Cook without moving the fillets until they release easily from the pan and the flesh is cooked about one-third of the way up the sides, 6 to 7 minutes. Flip the fillets and cook on the second side until golden, 2 to 3 minutes (the center will still be slightly pink), a minute longer if you prefer your fish fully cooked.

Dollop a mound of the pea puree on each serving plate and top with a fish fillet, browned side up. Drizzle each serving with a bit of the chile oil and serve (see Hint).

HINT HINT ◆ For a restaurant-style presentation, cook the salmon with the skin on until cracker-crisp, remove the skin and drizzle the salmon with chile oil, then place the skin back across the fillet at a jaunty angle.

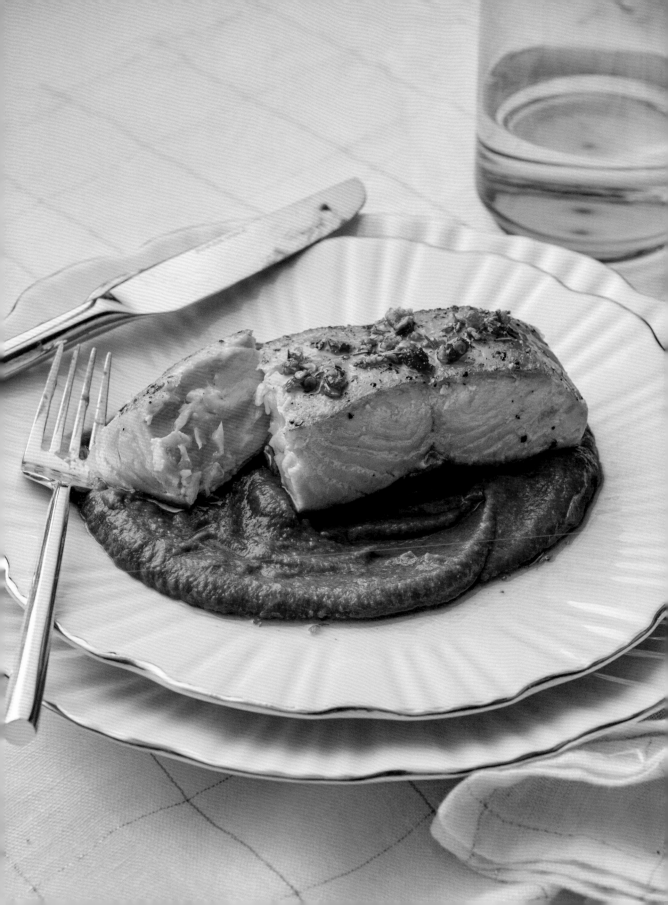

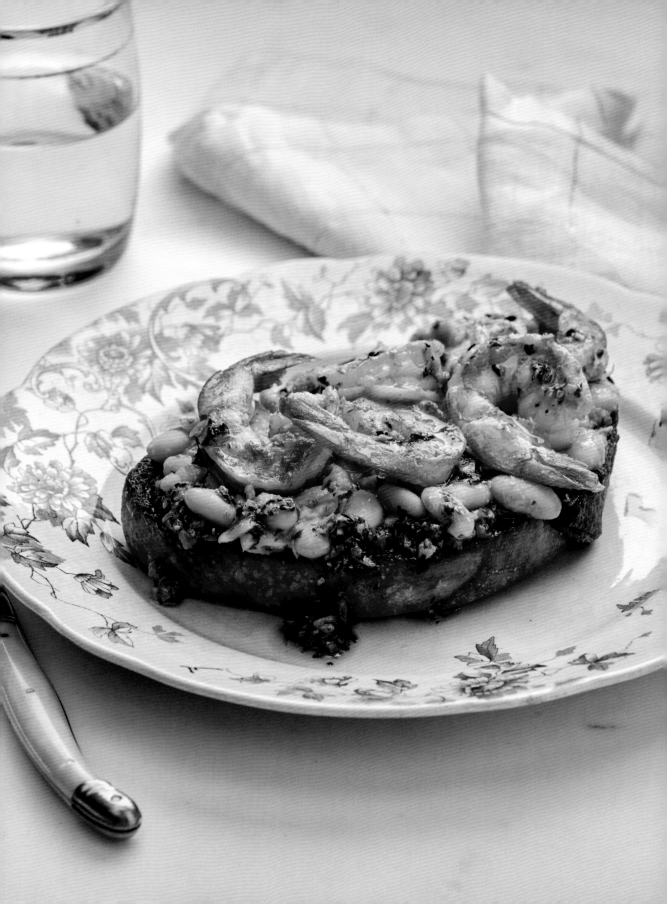

Lemony Shrimp AND Beans

ON TOAST

I like to find ways to lighten up beans and turn them into something other than a soup or a chili. Here they extend a pricier ingredient like shrimp and add a silky note to the sauce. This is a super-fast, super-homey, super-comforting way to eat.

Serves

4

2 tablespoons extra-virgin olive oil, plus more for drizzling

3 garlic cloves, smashed and peeled

2 anchovy fillets

1 pound extra-large shrimp, peeled and deveined, tails on

½ teaspoon GDL Seasoned Salt [page 48]

½ cup dry white wine

2 (15-ounce) cans cannellini beans, partially drained

1½ teaspoons kosher salt

1½ cups Parmesan Chicken Broth [page 64] or low-sodium store-bought chicken broth, plus a 2-inch piece Parmigiano-Reggiano rind

Grated zest and juice of 1 lemon

¼ cup chopped fresh flat-leaf Italian parsley

4 slices sourdough bread, toasted

½ cup Kale Salsa Verde [page 54]

In a medium skillet, heat the oil over medium heat. Add the garlic and anchovies and cook, stirring, until the anchovies have melted into the oil and the garlic is golden. Discard the garlic.

Add the shrimp to the skillet in a single layer and sprinkle with the seasoned salt. Increase the heat to high and cook the shrimp on just one side until the tails are turning pink and the undersides are browned around the edges, about 4 minutes. Transfer the shrimp to a bowl.

Add the wine to the skillet and cook for a minute, scraping the bottom of the pan with a wooden spoon. Add the beans, kosher salt, and broth (use a bit of the broth to rinse out any bean residue from the can and add it to the pan). Reduce the heat to medium and simmer until the liquid in the pan has thickened to the consistency of heavy cream, 5 to 10 minutes, using a fork to mash a few of the beans into the liquid. Stir in the lemon zest and juice, parsley, and the shrimp with any juices from the bowl and stir together for a minute or two to rewarm the shrimp and to cook through.

Spread each piece of toast with 2 tablespoons of the salsa verde and place in a shallow bowl. Spoon the shrimp and beans on the toasts, drizzling with the pan juices and a bit of olive oil. Serve hot.

Crunchy Baked Sole

WITH CAPERS

I've been able to convert quite a few fish haters into fish lovers with this dish, a cross between a piccata and an oreganata that bakes in the oven and makes its own lemony sauce. Serve this over rice, with a bit of bread, or on a bed of greens.

Serves

4

◆

1 lemon, thinly sliced

4 Dover sole or other thin white fish fillets

¾ teaspoon kosher salt

¼ cup dry white wine

2 tablespoons fresh lemon juice

¼ cup drained capers

3 tablespoons unsalted butter, cut into small bits

½ cup Garlicky Bread Crumbs [page 47]

¼ cup freshly grated Parmigiano-Reggiano cheese

1 tablespoon extra-virgin olive oil

Preheat the oven to 450°F.

In a large ovenproof skillet or baking dish large enough to hold the fish in a single layer with a little space between the fillets, arrange the lemon slices. Season the fish with the salt and arrange in the skillet or baking dish. Add the wine, lemon juice, and capers to the pan, then distribute the butter among the fillets.

In a small bowl, stir the bread crumbs together with the cheese. Sprinkle the crumb mixture onto the fish and drizzle with the oil.

Roast the fish until the crumbs are deep golden brown, 8 to 10 minutes. (If your fillets are very thin you may want to start checking them for doneness after 6 minutes or so.) Serve drizzled with the pan juices.

Roasted Branzino
WITH Melted Leeks AND Fennel

In Italy, smaller fish like branzino or sea bass are often stuffed with vegetables or herbs and served whole, which gives the flesh so much flavor while keeping it moist. In my experience, though, Americans are much less comfortable confronting a fish with head, tail, and fins intact, so I have adapted this recipe to use fillets, which your fishmonger can make from the whole fish for you. If you'd like to try cooking a whole fish, though, this is an excellent entry point! Just stuff the cavity with the parsley, lemon, and fennel fronds and roast as directed.

Serves
4

2 tablespoons extra-virgin olive oil

2 large leeks, white parts only, halved lengthwise and thinly sliced

1 large fennel bulb (stalks removed and fronds reserved for garnish), halved lengthwise and thinly sliced

2 teaspoons kosher salt

4 branzino fillets (5 to 6 ounces each) or 2 whole branzino (about 1 pound each)

4 stalks fresh flat-leaf Italian parsley

1 lemon, thinly sliced

1 cup Kale Salsa Verde (page 54)

Preheat the oven to 450°F.

In a large ovenproof skillet, heat the oil over medium-high heat. Add the leeks and fennel, season with 1½ teaspoons of the salt, and sauté until the fennel has softened and the leeks are silky, about 12 minutes, adding a bit of water to the pan if the mixture begins to stick. Leave the vegetables in the skillet and set aside.

Place the fish fillets on a work surface skin side down. Season with the remaining ½ teaspoon salt, then top 2 of the fillets with some fennel fronds, the parsley stalks, and 2 or 3 lemon slices. Top each with a second fish fillet, skin side up, and press gently to sandwich the filling between them. Arrange the fish packages atop the fennel and leek mixture.

Roast in the oven until the fish is cooked through and the flesh of the bottom fillet flakes easily with a fork, 17 to 20 minutes.

To serve, transfer the fish fillets to a serving platter, opening them up like a book and discarding the lemon and herb stalks. Spoon the vegetable mixture around the fillets. Drizzle with a generous amount of the salsa verde, top with chopped fennel fronds, and pass additional salsa verde at the table.

Seared Scallops

WITH PARMESAN BASIL BUTTER

I serve scallops fairly often because my partner, Shane, really adores them. I love how fast they are to make, because their delicate flavor really shines brightest when you do as little as possible to them—just a dab of compound butter from the freezer is all it takes. Try to buy really fresh scallops that have not previously been frozen, which are just so much sweeter.

Serves

4

❖

2 large russet potatoes,
peeled and quartered

1 garlic clove

3 teaspoons kosher salt

6 tablespoons Parmesan Basil Butter
(page 56), frozen solid

3 tablespoons extra-virgin olive oil

2 tablespoons unsalted butter

12 to 16 large sea scallops, side
muscles removed (see Hint)

HINT HINT ❖ Scallops vary a lot in size; I find 3 of the extra-large ones often labeled diver scallops enough for a serving, but if the "large" scallops in your store are not all that large, you will want to allow 4 or even 5 per person.

In a large saucepan of water, combine the potatoes and garlic and bring to a boil over high heat. When the water boils, add 1 teaspoon of the salt, reduce the heat to medium, and boil until the potatoes can be easily pierced with the tip of a knife, about 20 minutes. Reserve 1 cup of the cooking water, then drain the potatoes and return to the pot to steam for a minute or two.

Use a potato masher to mash the potatoes fairly smooth. Grate 4 tablespoons of the basil butter into the pot, add 1 tablespoon of the oil, and continue to mash until the potatoes are very light and smooth, adding the cooking water by ¼ cup to achieve your preferred consistency. Add 1 teaspoon salt and stir with a rubber spatula until incorporated. Keep warm while you cook the scallops.

In a large skillet, heat the unsalted butter and the remaining 2 tablespoons oil together over medium-high heat. Pat the scallops dry with paper towels, then sprinkle lightly with the remaining 1 teaspoon salt. When the butter mixture is very hot (don't jump the gun!), add the scallops in a single layer, allowing a bit of room between them. Cook the scallops without moving until the bottoms are deep golden brown, about 3 minutes. If they stick to the pan when you try to turn them, they are not ready; when the surface is seared, they will release easily.

Flip the scallops and cook on the second side until they are just cooked through, 1 or 2 minutes. Remove from the heat.

Mound some of the potatoes on each serving plate and arrange 3 or 4 scallops on top. Grate the remaining 2 tablespoons basil butter over the scallops, drizzle with some of the pan juices, and serve immediately.

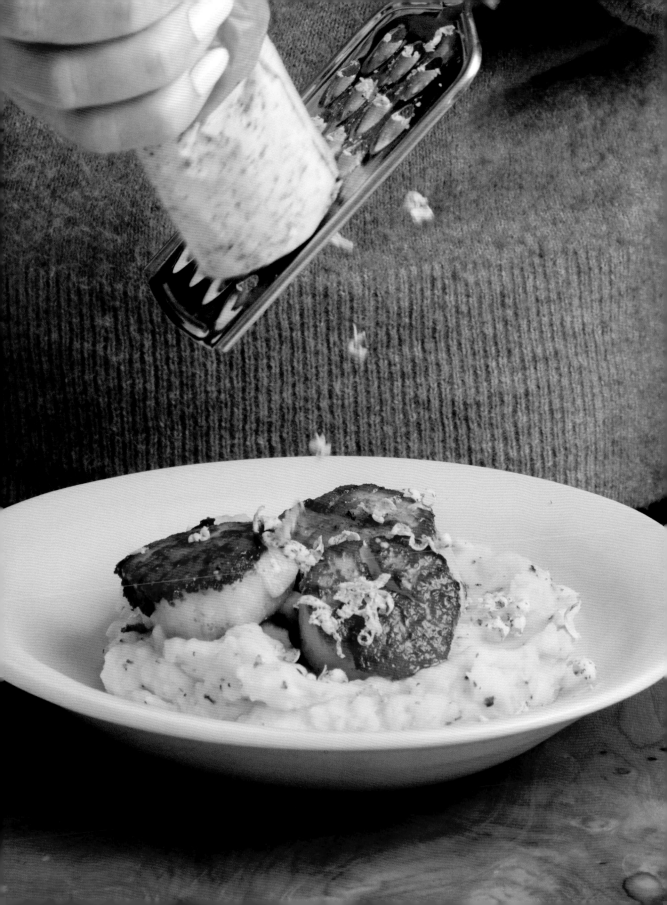

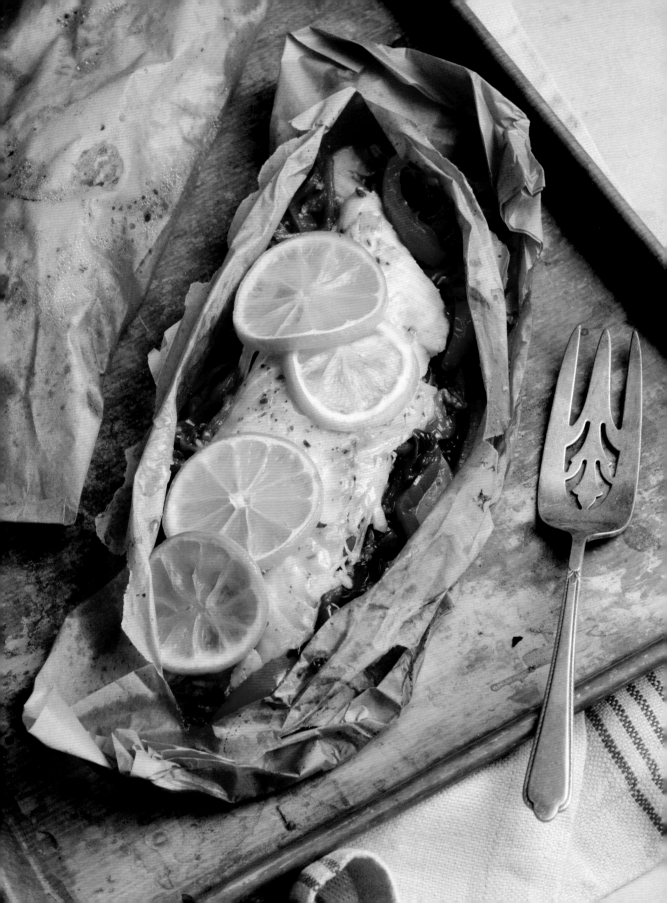

Snapper Packets
WITH **Potatoes** AND **Peperonata**

I'm not sure why people get intimidated by cooking "en papillote," a fancy way of saying in a parchment packet. The simple folding technique looks more complicated than it actually is and it creates a steamy environment that keeps the fish from drying out and lets the aromatics perfume the fish as it cooks. For this recipe, you can prepare all the components ahead of time, assemble the packets, then pop them in the oven just before you are ready to serve.

Serves
4

◆

4 small Yukon Gold potatoes

2 cups Peperonata (page 59)

2 large or 4 small red snapper or sea bass fillets (about 1½ pounds total)

1 teaspoon GDL Seasoned Salt (page 48)

1 lemon, sliced

¼ cup Garlicky Bread Crumbs (page 47)

Preheat the oven to 400°F.

In a saucepan of well-salted boiling water, cook the potatoes until nearly tender, about 6 minutes. Drain and when cool enough to handle, cut into ¼-inch-thick slices.

Place two 24-inch pieces of parchment paper on your work surface and crease each in the middle lengthwise. Arrange half the potato slices just to one side of the crease, creating a bed of potatoes on each piece of parchment about the size of a fish fillet. (If you are using smaller fish fillets, you can fit 2 end to end in each parchment packet.)

Spread half the peperonata over each bed of potatoes, then place the fish fillet(s) on top. Sprinkle the fish with the seasoned salt, then arrange a few lemon slices on each fillet.

To make each packet, fold the parchment paper over the fish and then, starting at the edge nearest you, fold and crimp the two layers of parchment together, making a series of small folds as you follow the contour of the fish. Place the sealed packets on a sheet pan.

Bake until the packets are puffed and browned, about 25 minutes.

Let cool for 5 minutes or so, then cut or tear open the packets to allow the steam to escape. With a sharp knife, cut each large fish fillet into 2 portions, cutting down through all the layers. Use a large spatula to transfer the fish, peppers, and potatoes to plates and serve with a sprinkle of bread crumbs.

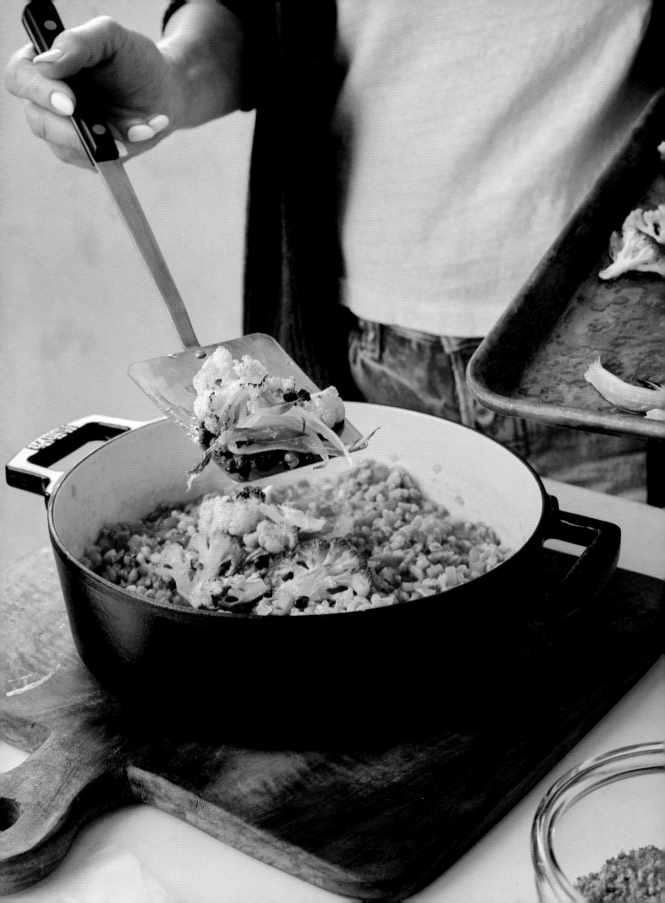

Seven

Meatless Mains

Because my mother

HAS BEEN A VEGETARIAN

———◆———

for most of her life and cooked that way for me and my siblings, eating a meal that isn't focused on meat or even fish (which she does eat occasionally) is nothing out of the ordinary for me. It doesn't have to be Meatless Monday or part of a New Year's resolution for me to skip meat for dinner once or twice a week, and because I never acquired the habit of stashing meat in the freezer, if I can't get to the store there are plenty of nights when I don't happen to have any to cook. At times like those, or if I just feel like eating something light, I turn to the pantry for a quick, filling meal.

Eggs often play a role in that scenario, as does rice or another grain like farro or polenta. Beyond that starting point, though, you should consider the dishes in this section as an invitation to improvisation. If you don't have the specific cheese, vegetable, or whatever that I recommend, use what you've got; it's what my mother did and what I now do for myself and Jade.

One caveat: Though none of these dishes features a significant serving of meat, they are not all strictly vegetarian. (If you are looking for completely vegetarian or vegan dishes, you will find plenty of recipes in this book that will fit the bill.) I do, for instance, use chicken broth in some of my risottos and there is a small amount of (nonvegetarian) anchovies in the bread crumbs that make the vegetable terrine so savory. You are welcome to eliminate or modify those elements to your needs if you observe a true vegetarian diet. Because I am an omnivore, I'd rather use those small amounts of animal products to add richness and depth than rely on a mountain of cheese to add flavor, hardly the healthier option, but you do you!

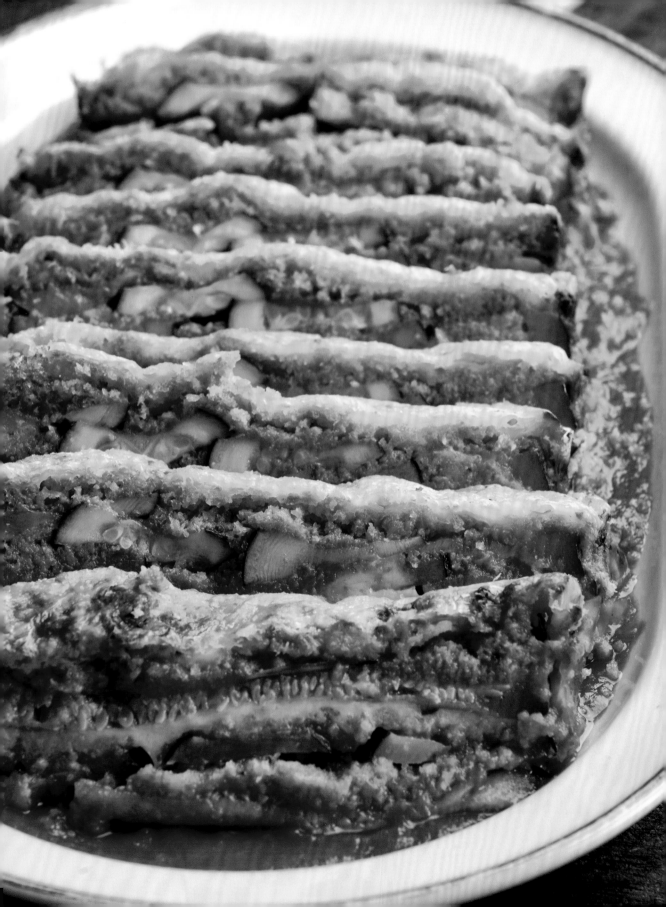

Zucchini Parmesan Terrine

Adding a few bread crumbs to a baked casserole of zucchini, mozzarella, and Parmesan gives it a firmer, sliceable texture that looks so pretty on the plate. Served in a puddle of sauce, this would also make an elegant first course for a fancy dinner.

Serves
6 TO 8

- 4 medium to large zucchini

- 1 tablespoon kosher salt

- 2 cups Simple Tomato Sauce [page 63], plus more for serving [optional]

- ⅓ cup Garlicky Bread Crumbs [page 47]

- ½ cup freshly grated Parmigiano-Reggiano cheese

- ½ cup grated mozzarella cheese

Preheat the oven to 425°F.

Trim tops and bottoms from the zucchini, and slice them lengthwise into ¼-inch strips. Arrange them on a kitchen towel and sprinkle on both sides with the salt. Cover with a second towel, then place a sheet pan on top and add a can or two to the pan to lightly press out some of the moisture from the zucchini. Let the zucchini drain for 15 minutes.

Spread ¼ cup of the tomato sauce in the bottom of a 9 × 5-inch loaf pan. Add a layer of zucchini, cutting the strips as needed to cover the sauce completely. Top with another ¼ cup sauce, then sprinkle with 1 tablespoon of the bread crumbs and 1 tablespoon of the Parmigiano. Repeat the layer, then add half the mozzarella.

Continue to layer in the zucchini, sauce, crumbs, and Parmigiano for four layers in total, ending with the remaining mozzarella. You will need to increase the amount of crumbs and sauce a bit for the third and fourth layers to cover the surface, as the pan will be wider near the top. Sprinkle the terrine with the remaining Parmigiano.

Bake until the top of the terrine is golden brown and bubbling around the edges, about 25 minutes.

Let the terrine cool for at least 15 minutes before slicing. Serve with additional sauce if desired.

Asparagus AND Pea Risotto

WITH FRIED EGG

I'm not sure why some people are intimidated by risotto, because the hardest part of the process is having the patience to stir, stir, and stir some more! Other than that, it requires minimal prep, can be made entirely with ingredients from the pantry, and always looks impressive. Topping a dish with a fried egg is common practice in Italy—Tuscan steak is a classic example—and here it adds protein and interest to this entirely vegetarian risotto. If it's a step too far, you can certainly leave it out.

Serves
4

6 cups Savory Vegetable Broth (page 65)

2-inch piece Parmigiano-Reggiano rind

½ pound asparagus, tough ends trimmed

4 tablespoons extra-virgin olive oil

2 shallots, 1 chopped, 1 thinly sliced

1½ cups Carnaroli or Arborio rice

1½ teaspoons kosher salt

1 cup dry white wine

1 cup frozen peas

2 tablespoons unsalted butter

½ cup freshly grated Parmigiano-Reggiano cheese

4 large eggs

In a saucepan, bring the broth and Parm rind to a simmer. Turn the heat to very low and keep warm.

Cut the asparagus into ½-inch pieces, keeping the flower ends whole and slicing them in half lengthwise. Set aside.

In a heavy-bottomed pan or small Dutch oven, heat 2 tablespoons of the oil over medium-high heat. Add the chopped shallot and cook until softened, about 2 minutes. Add the rice and toast it, stirring frequently, until the grains are uniformly white and opaque, about 2 minutes. Season with ½ teaspoon of the salt. Add the wine, bring to a simmer, and cook until the rice has almost completely absorbed the liquid, 3 to 4 minutes.

At this point, begin to add the warm broth to the pan 1 cup at a time. Keep the liquid at a simmer and stir the risotto frequently, waiting until each addition of broth has been mostly absorbed before adding more. Keep stirring and adding broth, up to 4 cups, until the grains of rice are just starting to become al dente, about 25 minutes in total.

While the risotto simmers, place the peas in a blender with 1 cup of the warm broth and ½ teaspoon salt. Puree until smooth. When the rice is nearly al dente, stir in the pea puree and the asparagus pieces. Continue to cook and stir the risotto until just tender.

Add the butter and cheese, stirring to combine. If the risotto is too thick (there should be a loose, creamy sauce around the grains of rice), stir in another ½ cup broth. Remove from the heat and keep warm.

CONTINUES

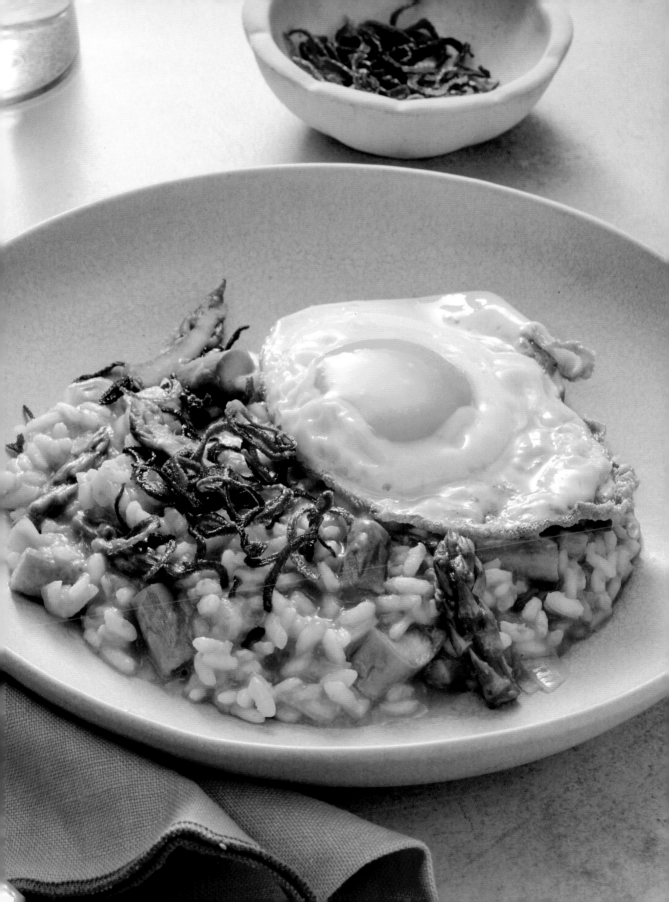

In a nonstick skillet, heat the remaining 2 tablespoons oil over medium-high heat. When the oil is hot, add the sliced shallots and sauté until frizzled, 2 to 4 minutes. Use a slotted spoon to transfer the shallots to a paper towel to drain.

Carefully crack the eggs into the same skillet. Fry, basting with the hot oil now and then, until the whites are set but the yolk is still runny, 4 or 5 minutes. (If you prefer the yolk more cooked, add a couple of tablespoons of water to the skillet, cover with a lid, and cook until the eggs are cooked to your liking.) Season with the remaining ½ teaspoon salt.

Stir the risotto, adding a tiny bit more broth if needed to loosen it. Spoon the risotto into shallow serving bowls and top each portion with an egg and a sprinkle of the frizzled shallots. Serve immediately.

Polenta WITH Braised Mushrooms

The more different kinds of mushrooms you use here, the more fun this is to eat, with lots of different tastes and textures. It may sound like a lot of mushrooms but remember, they cook down a ton. I've kept the polenta pretty simple, so as not to take away from the savory, meaty flavors of the mushrooms, but if you want, stir in up to ¾ cup of grated Parmigiano or pecorino when the polenta has finished cooking.

Serves
4

1 ounce dried porcini mushrooms

2 tablespoons extra-virgin olive oil

2 tablespoons unsalted butter

1 shallot, finely chopped

2 pounds mixed mushrooms, trimmed and sliced

1½ teaspoons kosher salt

1 tablespoon tomato paste

½ teaspoon chopped fresh rosemary

4 fresh thyme sprigs

½ cup dry red wine

2 cups Parmesan Chicken Broth (page 64), Savory Vegetable Broth (page 65), or store-bought low-sodium chicken or vegetable broth

2 cups baby kale or baby spinach

FOR THE POLENTA

¾ cup quick-cooking polenta

3 tablespoons unsalted butter

1 teaspoon kosher salt, plus more to taste

¼ cup mascarpone cheese

¼ cup chopped fresh flat-leaf Italian parsley

Place the dried porcini in a glass measuring cup and add about a cup of hot water, or enough to cover. Set aside to hydrate for 15 minutes. Reserving the soaking liquid, drain the softened mushrooms and chop into small pieces.

In a large sauté pan, heat the oil and butter over medium-high heat. When the butter melts, add the shallot and cook until beginning to soften, about 2 minutes. Add the fresh mushrooms and toss to coat with the fat, then spread them over the pan in a single layer. Let the mushrooms cook without stirring until browned on the bottom, 5 or 6 minutes. Stir and brown for another 3 minutes.

Season the mushrooms with the salt, then add the tomato paste, rosemary, and thyme and stir to combine. Add the wine and cook until it has mostly evaporated, about 3 minutes, scraping the bottom of the pan with a wooden spoon.

Strain about three-quarters of the mushroom soaking liquid into the pan, then add the broth and the chopped porcini. Bring the liquid to a boil, then reduce the heat to low, cover, and cook for 5 minutes.

Uncover, increase the heat to medium, and stir in the greens. Cook until the greens are tender and the liquid has reduced by half, 5 to 8 minutes.

Meanwhile, make the polenta: In a large saucepan, bring 3½ cups water to a boil. Whisk in the polenta, butter, and salt and cook, stirring frequently, until thickened, about 5 minutes. Taste for salt, then whisk in the mascarpone.

Mound the polenta in four shallow bowls and top with the mushrooms. Sprinkle with the parsley and serve.

Tomato Soup Risotto

Think of this as an Italian version of grilled cheese with tomato soup, except it's made fresh, not out of a can. It's just the thing I want to hunker down with on a rainy weekend afternoon when I need a big, warm hug of a meal.

Serves
4

2 tablespoons extra-virgin olive oil

3 tablespoons unsalted butter

1 shallot, chopped

2 garlic cloves, smashed and peeled

½ teaspoon kosher salt

1 (11-ounce) jar datterini tomatoes or 1 (15-ounce) can cherry tomatoes, drained

1 cup Carnaroli or Arborio rice

½ cup dry white wine

1 cup Savory Vegetable Broth (page 65) or low-sodium store-bought vegetable broth

¼ cup mascarpone cheese

1 cup freshly grated Parmigiano-Reggiano cheese, plus more (optional) for serving

2 tablespoons chopped fresh chives (optional)

In a medium Dutch oven, heat the oil and 1 tablespoon of the butter together over medium-high heat. When the butter has melted, add the shallot, garlic, and salt and cook until the shallot is beginning to soften, about 1 minute. Reduce the heat to medium.

Add the drained tomatoes to the pan and crush them a bit with a wooden spoon. Cook, stirring often until the tomatoes are all smashed and coated in the flavorful oil, about 3 minutes. Add the rice and stir until the tomato liquid is fully absorbed, about 3 minutes. Stir in the wine and simmer until it is fully absorbed, another 2 minutes. Add the broth and cook, stirring often, until it is almost entirely absorbed, about 5 minutes.

Add 1¼ cups water and cook, continuing to stir often to prevent the rice from sticking, until the rice is creamy and fluid but still a bit al dente, another 7 to 10 minutes. If it is too thick or still too al dente, add another ¼ cup water. Remove from the heat and stir in the remaining 2 tablespoons butter, the mascarpone, and the Parmigiano.

Spoon into shallow bowls. If desired, sprinkle with the chives and more Parmigiano and serve.

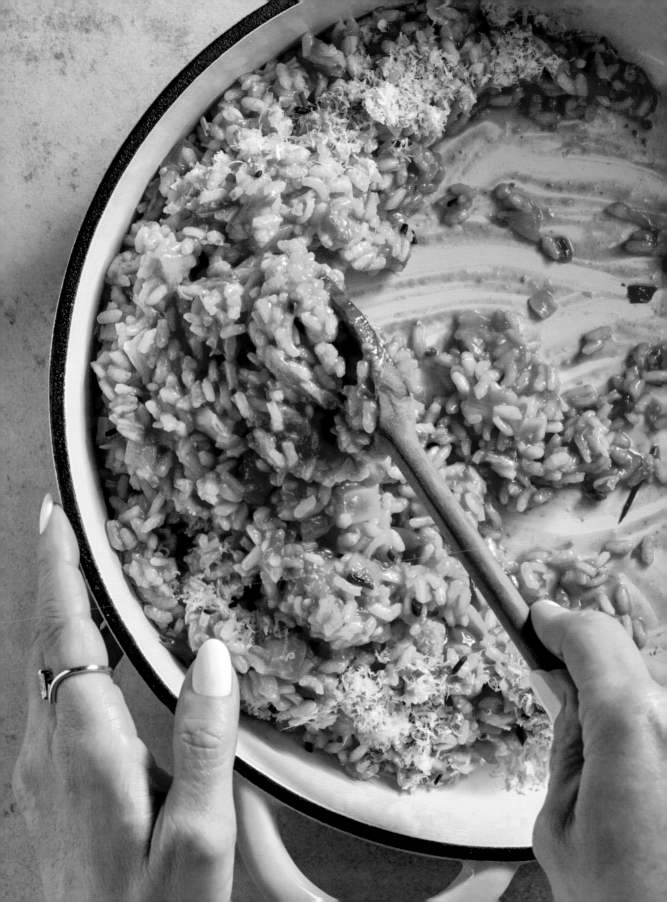

Loaded Baked Potato

WITH CAPONATA

Caponata is another versatile vegetable relish that could easily have made it into my condiment essentials, although it doesn't have quite as long a shelf life as the others. If you are missing one or two of the ingredients (or just don't love raisins), don't let that stop you from giving it a try. There are enough tastes and textures here that they won't be missed.

Serves

2

2 russet potatoes (8 to 10 ounces each), scrubbed

2 teaspoons extra-virgin olive oil

FOR THE CAPONATA

¼ cup extra-virgin olive oil

1 celery stalk, chopped

1 medium eggplant, unpeeled, cut into ½-inch chunks

1¼ teaspoons kosher salt, plus more to taste

1 red bell pepper, cut into ½-inch pieces

1 medium onion, chopped

1 (14.5-ounce) can diced tomatoes, undrained

3 tablespoons raisins

½ teaspoon dried Sicilian oregano

¼ teaspoon freshly ground black pepper, plus more to taste

¼ cup red wine vinegar

2 teaspoons sugar

1 tablespoon drained capers

2 tablespoons chopped fresh flat-leaf Italian parsley

Preheat the oven to 350°F.

Rub the potatoes all over with the 2 teaspoons oil and place directly on the oven rack to bake until they give when squeezed gently, about 1 hour.

Meanwhile, make the caponata: In a large heavy skillet, heat the ¼ cup oil over medium heat. Add the celery and sauté for 2 minutes. Add the eggplant and cook until the eggplant pieces are beginning to soften, about 2 minutes. Season with ½ teaspoon of the salt. Add the bell pepper and onion and cook, stirring fairly frequently, for 5 minutes.

Stir in the diced tomatoes with their juices, the raisins, the oregano, the remaining ¾ teaspoon salt, and the black pepper. Bring the mixture to a simmer over medium-low heat and cook, stirring now and then, until the flavors blend and the mixture thickens, about 20 minutes.

Stir in the vinegar, sugar, capers, and more salt and black pepper to taste if needed.

Slit open the tops of the potatoes and pinch the ends toward the middle to expose the flesh. Spoon the hot caponata into the potatoes, sprinkle with the parsley, and serve hot.

Skillet Eggs

WITH BREAD CRUMBS

Eggs are the ultimate clutch ingredient for those nights when you just need to throw something together without thinking about it too much, using things you already have on hand. This super simple dish is inspired by one of my culinary heroes, the late Judy Rodgers of San Francisco's Zuni Café. If you have a supply of garlicky bread crumbs on hand, this is ready in less than 10 minutes, but even if you have to make the crumbs from scratch, it won't even take a half hour. Don't be tempted to substitute pecorino for the Parm in this dish, as it will be too salty.

Serves
2 TO 4

1 cup Garlicky Bread Crumbs (page 47; see Hint)

½ cup freshly grated Parmigiano-Reggiano cheese

4 teaspoons extra-virgin olive oil, plus more for drizzling

4 large eggs

Kosher salt

3 cups baby arugula or baby spinach

Juice of ½ lemon

Stir the crumbs and Parmigiano together in a 12-inch nonstick skillet with a lid. Set over medium-low heat and cook for about 2 minutes, stirring often, to warm the crumbs. Use a silicone spatula to make 4 pockets in the crumbs and drizzle 1 teaspoon of the oil into each space. Crack an egg into each pocket and sprinkle the egg with a small pinch of salt. Cover the pan and cook, still over medium-low heat, until the eggs are just barely set and the cheese has melted.

Toss the greens with the lemon juice and a pinch or two of salt. Mound the greens in shallow serving bowls. Use a plastic spatula or other nonstick-safe implement to divide the skillet contents into 2 to 4 portions and slide each portion onto the mounds of greens. Drizzle everything with a bit of oil and serve.

HINT HINT ◆ If you don't have premade Garlicky Bread Crumbs on hand, this is a great time to make a batch. Prepare according to the recipe on page 47, being sure to use a nonstick skillet with a lid, and set aside 1 cup for future recipes, leaving the rest in the skillet and proceeding as above.

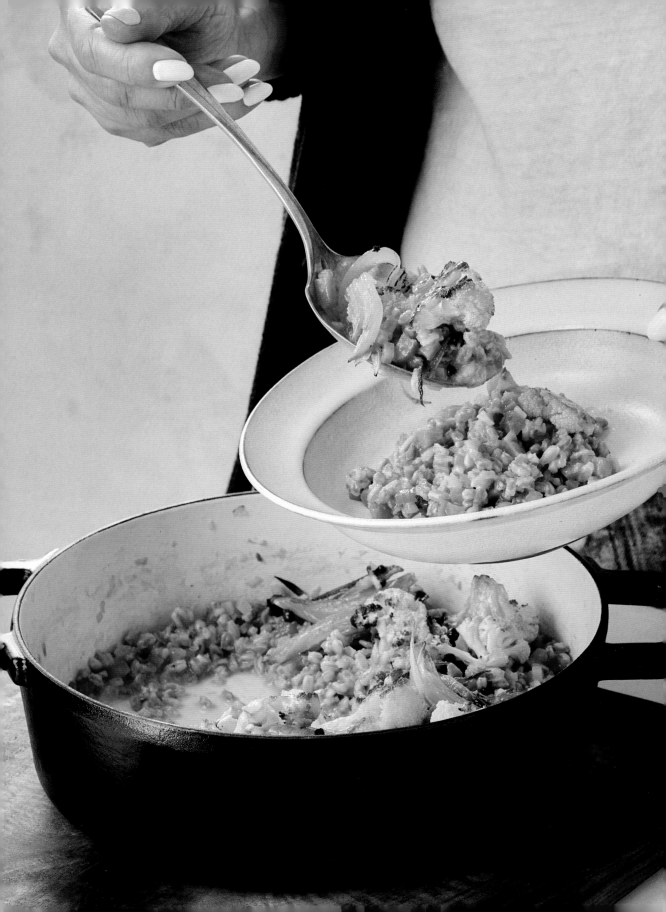

Cauliflower Farrotto

WITH ONIONS AND CAPERS

It's a bit of a cheat to call this a farrotto, because it bakes in the oven rather than being cooked on the stovetop and it's not as creamy as farro that you cook and stir and cook and stir and so on. On the other hand, you only need to stir it once or twice, a fair trade-off as far as I'm concerned. Since the oven is already on, it's so easy to caramelize some veggies to top the tender grains. I've used cauliflower, but butternut squash would be good here, as would broccoli or even green peas.

Serves
4 TO 6

FOR THE FARROTTO

2 tablespoons extra-virgin olive oil

1 shallot, finely chopped

1 small carrot, peeled and finely chopped

1 small celery stalk, finely chopped

2 garlic cloves, finely chopped

1 cup pearled farro

½ cup dry white wine

2½ cups Savory Vegetable Broth (page 65) or low-sodium store-bought vegetable broth

1 teaspoon kosher salt

2 tablespoons unsalted butter

¾ cup freshly grated pecorino cheese

FOR THE CARAMELIZED VEGETABLES

½ head cauliflower, sliced crosswise about ⅓ inch thick

1 onion, halved and sliced ¼ inch thick

¾ teaspoon GDL Seasoned Salt (page 48)

1½ tablespoons extra-virgin olive oil

2 tablespoons drained capers

2 to 3 tablespoons Garlicky Bread Crumbs (page 47)

Position two racks in the lower and upper third of the oven and preheat the oven to 425°F.

Make the farrotto: In an ovenproof skillet, heat the oil over medium-high heat. Add the shallot, carrot, and celery and cook until the vegetables are fairly soft, about 8 minutes. Add the garlic and stir for another minute. Stir in the farro and cook for 2 minutes to toast the grains, then stir in the wine. Cook until the wine has been absorbed, 1 to 2 minutes, then add the broth and kosher salt.

Transfer the skillet to the lower rack in the oven and bake the farro, uncovered, until the liquid has been absorbed and the grains are tender, about 30 minutes, stirring once or twice and adding more broth if the pan starts to look dry. Stir in the butter and the pecorino.

Meanwhile, prepare the caramelized vegetables: Arrange the cauliflower slices on a sheet pan, scattering any random pieces around the slices. Spread the onion slices over the cauliflower and sprinkle all with the seasoned salt. Drizzle with the oil.

Roast on the top rack until nice and caramelized, about 40 minutes, turning the vegetables with a metal spatula after about 25 minutes. Sprinkle with the capers.

Top the farrotto with the caramelized cauliflower, onion, and caper mixture. Sprinkle with the bread crumbs and serve.

Baked Egg Crepe Casserole

I have such warm, nostalgic feelings about this dish, which was a go-to for my mother when the day got away from her and she didn't have time to shop for dinner. Since we always had eggs, cheese, and tomato sauce around, it was a no-brainer to whip up a batch of these thin egg crepes and wrap up whatever leftover bits she found in the fridge with a pinch of cheese for an Italian version of enchiladas. I loved it then and I love it today when I find myself in the same nothing-to-make predicament!

Serves
4 OR 5

❧

6 large eggs

½ cup freshly grated Parmigiano-Reggiano cheese

1½ teaspoons kosher salt

8 to 10 teaspoons extra-virgin olive oil

2½ cups Simple Tomato Sauce [page 63] or Calabrian Pomodoro [page 61]

1½ cups cooked vegetables, such as asparagus, broccoli rabe, chard, spinach, mushrooms, or a combination

1½ cups grated mozzarella or provolone cheese, or a mixture of the two

Preheat the oven to 400°F.

In a medium bowl, beat the eggs, Parmigiano, and salt together with a fork until well combined.

Place a 10-inch nonstick skillet over medium heat. When the pan is hot, add 1 teaspoon of the oil and swirl to coat the surface. Add about 3 tablespoons of the egg mixture to the pan, swirling to coat the bottom evenly. Cook the crepe without disturbing it for about 3 minutes, or until the top looks set and nearly dry. Use a silicone spatula to lift the edges of the crepe to loosen, then flip and cook on the second side for a minute. Move the finished crepe to a plate and repeat with the remaining oil and eggs to make 8 or 9 more crepes.

Spread 1½ cups of the tomato sauce in the bottom of a 9 × 13-inch baking dish. One at a time, place the crepes on a work surface, add about 3 tablespoons of the veggies and sprinkle with about 1 tablespoon of the cheese. Carefully roll up the crepe and place in the baking dish, seam side down. When you have filled all the crepes, spoon the remaining tomato sauce over the crepes and sprinkle with the remaining cheese.

Bake until the sauce is bubbling, about 20 minutes. Serve hot.

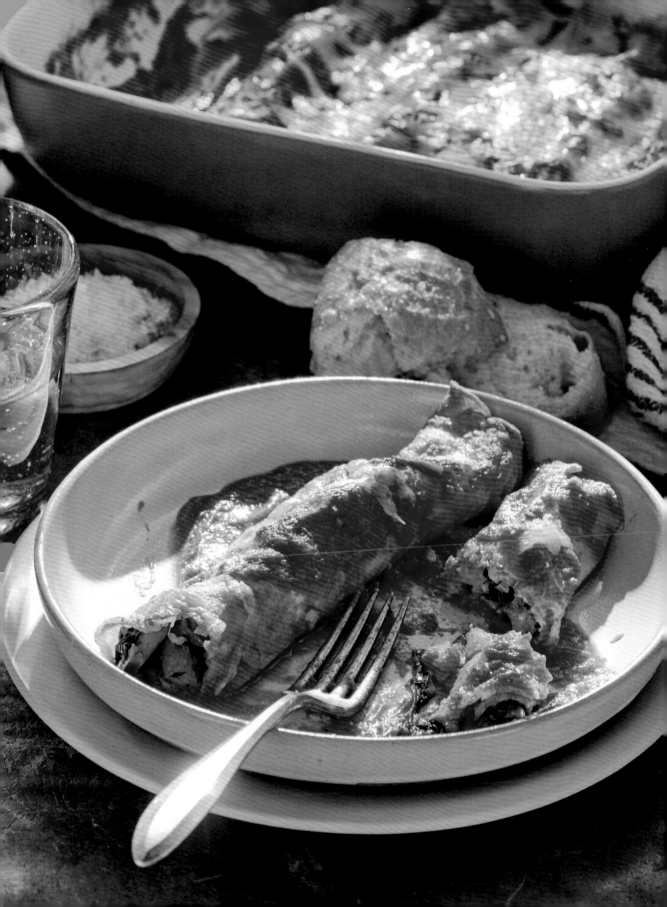

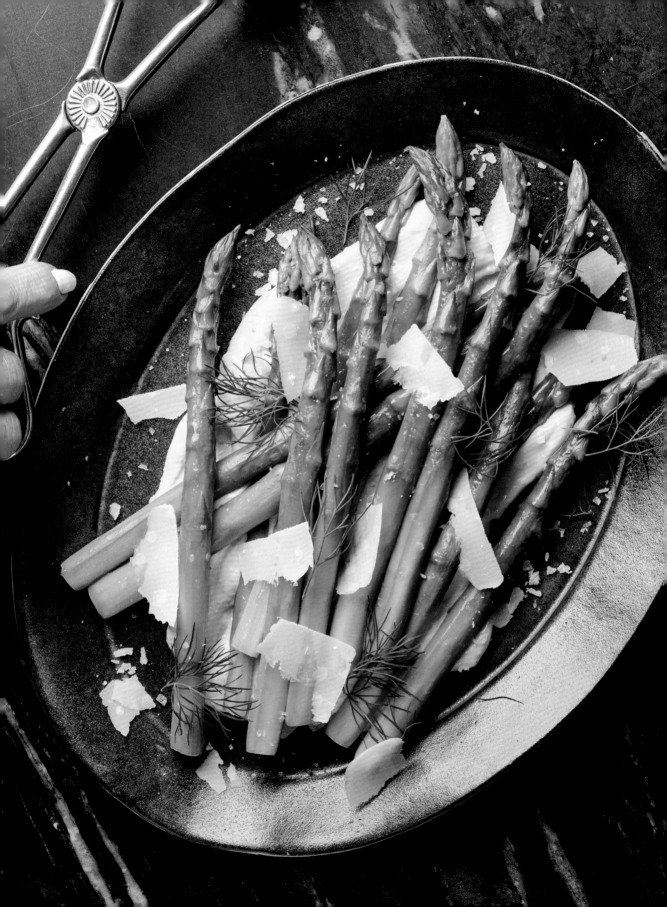

Eight — —

Sides

Pan-Fried Zucchini
with ANCHOVIES AND CAPERS 225

———

Thick Asparagus
with CAESAR AIOLI 226

———

Crispy Smashed Veggies
with Parm 229

———

Green Beans
with FRESH MINT AND GARLIC 230

———

Sautéed Swiss Chard
with Yellow Cherry Tomatoes 233

———

Roasted Broccolini
with SICILIAN PESTO 234

———

Tomatoes Gratinata 235

———

Sicilian Potato Salad 236

———

Spicy Lentils
with Kale 238

———

Creamy Cannellini Beans 239

———

Warm Farro
with Mushrooms
AND Brussels Sprouts 240

———

Grilled Artichokes
with GREEN OLIVE RELISH 241

———

Whenever I get a
NEW COOKBOOK,

I always turn immediately to the side dish chapter because that tends to be where you find the greatest concentration of vegetable recipes, and I can never get enough vegetables. I rarely plan a menu that doesn't include at *least* two vegetable dishes, often with a side salad to boot. Given how central vegetables are to my diet, it's almost a misnomer to call these dishes "sides," because this is where I spend a lot of time eating, and it's where I consume most of my calories. In a way, the meat and fish recipes are the side dishes!

Whatever you choose to call them, though, vegetables are the backbone of any meal I make. The recipes here are some I consider particularly versatile, as they pair with a wide variety of dishes, can be mixed and matched with one another, and in the case of the starchier options like the beans and lentils, are great building blocks for simple dinners.

Several of these recipes, like the grilled artichokes or the asparagus with an indulgent aioli dressing, would make a light but lovely first course. If you are entertaining, you might also consider making your own antipasto spread by assembling three or four veggie options (served warm or at room temperature) and allowing everyone to serve themselves. It's a particularly appealing way to encourage everyone at your table to make vegetables a bigger part of their diet.

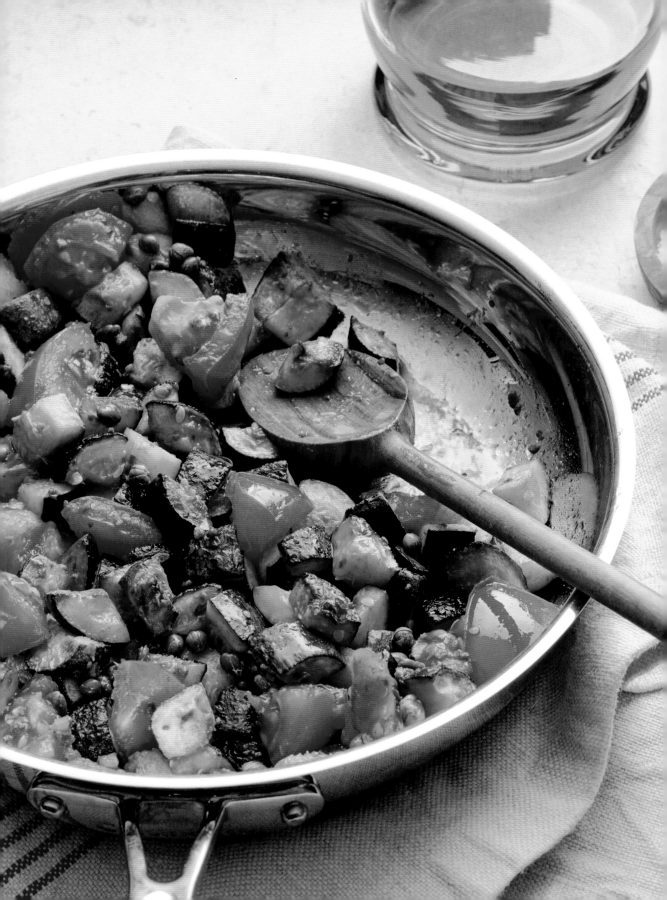

Pan-Fried Zucchini

WITH ANCHOVIES AND CAPERS

Zucchini doesn't get the love in this country that it does elsewhere, and Italians definitely make the most of it all summer long. It stores well in the fridge, soaks up lots of flavors, and can be served raw, lightly sautéed, or cooked to a velvety soft consistency, which makes it a very versatile vegetable to have in your crisper. Next to the Spaghetti Chitarra with Zucchini, Lemon, and Shrimp [page 138], this is one of my favorite ways to serve it; a healthy dose of anchovy, capers, Parmesan, and herbs definitely put the idea that zucchini is too bland to rest!

Serves
6

3 tablespoons extra-virgin olive oil

3 medium zucchini, quartered lengthwise and cut into ¾-inch pieces

½ teaspoon kosher salt

4 anchovy fillets, finely chopped

1 medium tomato, cored and diced

2 tablespoons drained capers

¼ teaspoon dried Sicilian oregano

¼ teaspoon red pepper flakes

1 tablespoon fresh lemon juice

¼ cup freshly grated Parmigiano-Reggiano cheese

2 tablespoons chopped fresh flat-leaf Italian parsley

In a large skillet, heat the oil over medium-high heat. Add the zucchini in a single layer and cook until deep golden brown on one side, about 4 minutes. Sprinkle with the salt, then turn the pieces and cook until browned on a second side, another 3 to 4 minutes. Use a slotted spoon to transfer the zucchini to a paper towel–lined plate to drain.

Add the anchovies to the oil remaining in the skillet and stir over medium heat, breaking them up with a wooden spoon until they have melted into the oil, a minute or two. Add the tomato, capers, oregano, pepper flakes, and lemon juice and stir to combine.

Just before serving, return the zucchini to the skillet and toss with the tomato mixture. Sprinkle with the Parmigiano and mix gently. Transfer to a serving bowl or platter, sprinkle with the chopped parsley, and serve.

Thick Asparagus

WITH CAESAR AIOLI

Having produce imported from around the world means that vegetables that were once considered seasonal are now available to us all year long. But even though it is easy to find asparagus any month of the year, nothing compares to the flavor of freshly harvested spears from the farmers' market in early spring. I especially like the big fat ones, which I think are milder and have a better texture. Simply steamed and served with a dollop of lemony, cheesy aioli, it's an Italian update on asparagus with hollandaise that would be ideal on an Easter table or with broiled salmon.

Serves
4

1½ pounds thick asparagus (about 16 fat spears)

2 tablespoons unsalted butter

½ teaspoon kosher salt

¾ cup Caesar Aioli (page 53)

Chunk of Parmigiano-Reggiano cheese, for shaving

Fennel fronds, for garnish (optional)

Trim off the woody bottom inch from the asparagus spears, then use a vegetable peeler to peel the bottom half of each spear.

Place the asparagus in a large skillet with the butter and ½ cup water. Bring the water to a boil, then reduce the heat to low, cover, and cook until the spears are tender when pierced with a knife, about 6 minutes.

Sprinkle the asparagus with the salt, increase the heat to high, and cook the asparagus, rolling to coat with the buttery pan juices, until the water has evaporated, about 2 minutes.

Spoon the aioli onto a serving platter and arrange the asparagus on top. Shave some fat ribbons of Parmigiano over it all and sprinkle with fennel fronds (if using). Serve warm or at room temperature.

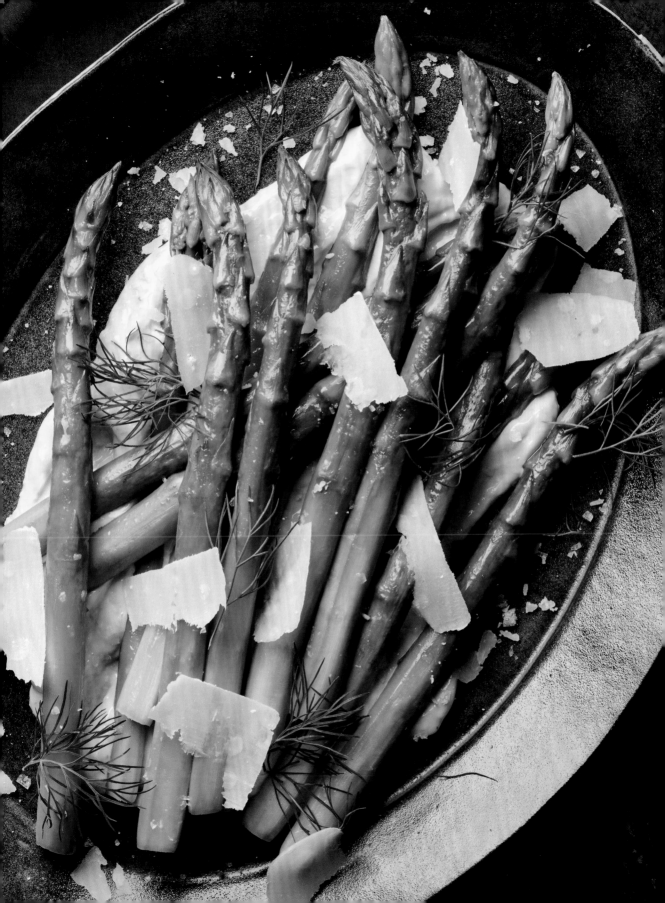

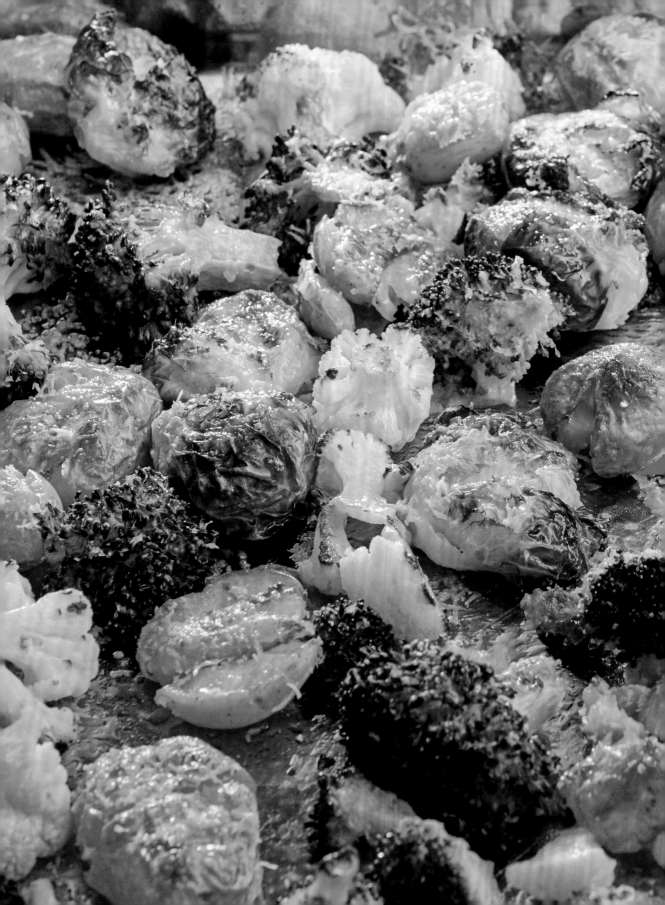

Crispy Smashed Veggies with Parm

I've learned I can get Jade to eat just about anything if it has a coating of crisp Parmesan. It doesn't really take a ton of cheese to turn "Ugh, broccoli again" into "More, please!" and I love taking the veggie battles off the table. That alone is worth the extra step of blanching the vegetables before they go in the oven. This side works as both starch and green, an added plus!

Serves
6

6 to 8 small Yukon Gold potatoes (about ½ pound total), halved

½ pound Brussels sprouts, trimmed

1 broccoli crown, cut into florets

½ head cauliflower, cut into 2-inch florets

4 tablespoons extra-virgin olive oil

1½ teaspoons kosher salt

½ cup freshly grated Parmigiano-Reggiano cheese

Position a rack in the top third of the oven and preheat the oven to 450°F.

Bring a large saucepan of salted water to a boil. Add the potatoes and cook for 6 minutes. Add the Brussels sprouts, broccoli, and cauliflower, return to a boil, and cook until the vegetables are nearly tender, another 4 minutes. Drain well.

Drizzle a sheet pan with 2 tablespoons of the oil. Spread the vegetables on the pan in a single layer. Using the heel of your hand or the bottom of a wine bottle, gently press down on the veggies to flatten them a bit. Drizzle with the remaining 2 tablespoons oil, sprinkle with the salt, and dust with the cheese.

Roast the vegetables until the cheese is golden and crisp, 12 to 15 minutes. Serve warm or at room temperature.

Green Beans

WITH FRESH MINT AND GARLIC

Maybe it's the associations with candy canes and toothpaste, but I find that a lot of cooks are dubious about using mint in the kitchen. That's a shame, because I absolutely love the freshness it contributes to all kinds of dishes, like basil [to which it is related botanically] but with a slightly sharper edge. Here it really wakes up a simple dish of green beans that might read a bit boring on the page but has loads of flavor on the plate. Don't undercook the beans; they should be closer to tender than crisp. This tastes best at room temperature.

Serves
4 TO 6

1 pound green beans, trimmed

2 tablespoons extra-virgin olive oil

Grated zest and juice of
½ large lemon

½ cup chopped fresh mint leaves,
plus a few whole leaves for garnish

¾ teaspoon kosher salt

¼ teaspoon freshly ground
black pepper

2 small garlic cloves, peeled

Bring a large pot of salted water to a boil. Add the beans and cook at a gentle boil until fairly tender, 6 to 8 minutes. Drain the beans and leave in the colander to cool to room temperature.

In a large bowl, combine the oil, lemon zest and juice, half the mint, the salt, and the pepper. Use a Microplane to grate the garlic directly into the bowl, then whisk the dressing thoroughly to combine.

Add the beans to the bowl, toss to coat with the dressing, and let stand at room temperature until ready to serve. Just before serving, add the remaining chopped and whole mint, toss, and serve.

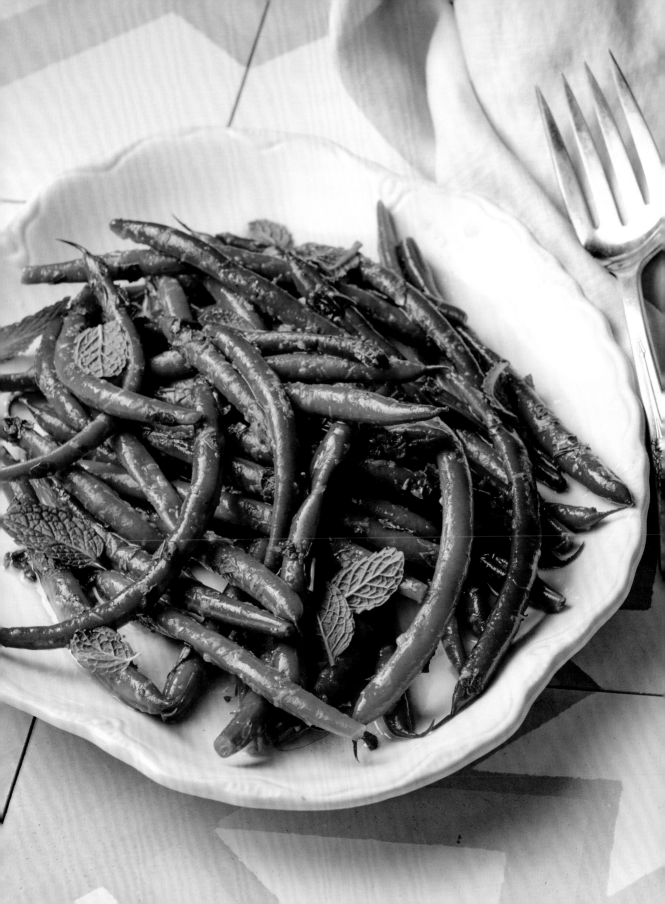

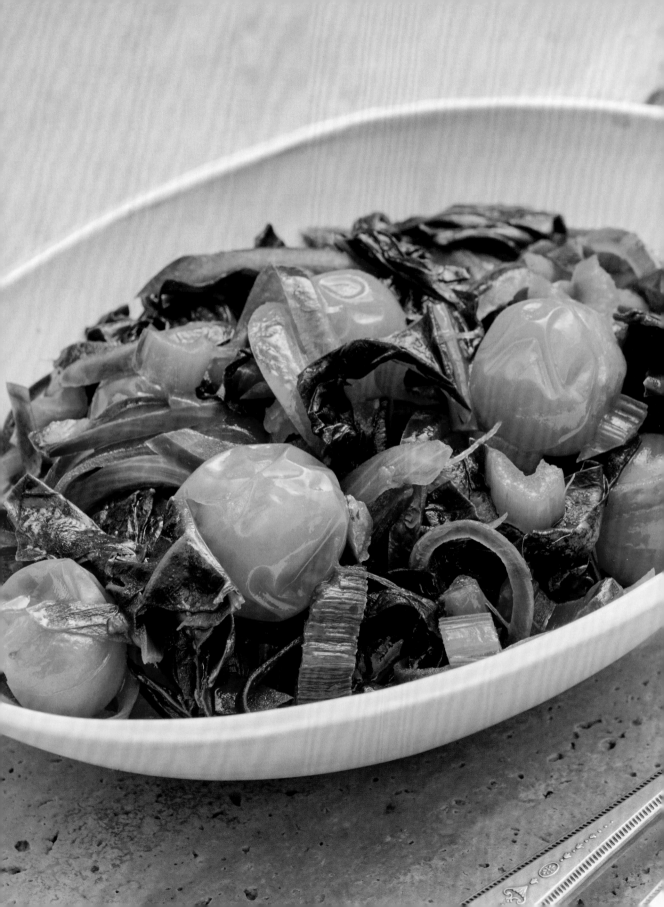

Sautéed Swiss Chard
WITH Yellow Cherry Tomatoes

Swiss chard is like spinach's gutsier big brother, and while it shares most of spinach's nutritional virtues, I think it holds up better to cooking without becoming soggy or mushy. I also love the way it looks growing in my garden, especially when I can find the rainbow variety. The stems are deliciously crunchy when sautéed, so don't toss them!

Serves
4

❖

1 bunch Swiss chard, preferably rainbow or red-stemmed

2 tablespoons extra-virgin olive oil

½ small red onion, thinly sliced

1 pint yellow cherry tomatoes, such as Sweet 100s

1 teaspoon kosher salt

¼ teaspoon red pepper flakes

2 tablespoons chicken broth or water

Separate the stems from the leaves of the chard and thinly slice the stems. Cut the leaves into 1-inch ribbons, then slice the ribbons crosswise into 2- to 3-inch pieces.

In a large skillet, heat the oil over medium heat. Add the sliced chard stems and the onion and sauté until softened, about 4 minutes. Add the tomatoes, sprinkle with ½ teaspoon of the salt, and the pepper flakes. Toss to coat, then stir in the chard leaves and broth. Cover the pan and cook until the chard leaves are wilted and the tomatoes start to wrinkle, about 7 minutes.

Sprinkle with the remaining ½ teaspoon salt and serve.

Roasted Broccolini WITH SICILIAN PESTO

If broccolini seems like it just came on the scene recently, that's because it did! It's actually a hybrid of two vegetables, regular broccoli and slender-stemmed Chinese broccoli, and the resulting plant has a tender stalk that is completely edible and doesn't need peeling. Jade prefers it to broccoli rabe because it is sweeter; I like that its flavor is less cabbage-y than standard broccoli. It takes well to roasting with virtually no prep!

Serves
4

2 bunches broccolini, trimmed

1 tablespoon extra-virgin olive oil

½ teaspoon kosher salt

¼ teaspoon freshly ground black pepper

½ cup Sicilian Pesto (page 60)

Preheat the oven to 425°F. Line a sheet pan with parchment paper.

Mound the broccolini on the sheet pan and drizzle with the oil, tossing to coat. Spread the spears in a single layer and sprinkle with the salt and pepper.

Roast the broccolini until it is deeply browned, almost charred in spots and the stems are tender when pierced with a knife, about 15 minutes.

Spoon the pesto onto a serving platter and arrange the broccolini on top (or vice versa if you prefer). Serve warm or at room temperature.

Tomatoes Gratinata

At the risk of sounding like a broken record, the more simply you cook, the more important the quality of your ingredients becomes. Sure, you can make this in January, using imported vine tomatoes, and it will be just fine. But make it at the height of summer with amazing, juicy tomatoes from a local farm stand, and the flavor will be off the charts.

Serves
4 TO 6

2 beefsteak or heirloom tomatoes

Kosher salt

1 cup Garlicky Bread Crumbs
[page 47]

½ cup freshly grated
Parmigiano-Reggiano cheese

1 tablespoon finely chopped fresh
flat-leaf Italian parsley

2 to 3 tablespoons extra-virgin
olive oil

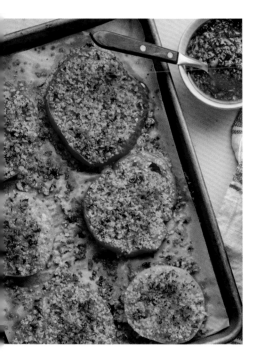

With a serrated knife, cut a ½-inch slice off the top and bottom of each tomato and reserve for another use. Cut each tomato into 2 or 3 slices about ¾ inch thick. Arrange the slices on a double layer of paper towels and sprinkle generously with salt. Let the tomatoes drain for 15 minutes.

While the tomatoes drain, position a rack in the upper third of the oven and preheat the oven to 450°F. Line a sheet pan with parchment paper.

Arrange the tomatoes on the prepared sheet pan in a single layer. Sprinkle with salt. In a small bowl, stir together the crumbs, cheese, and parsley. Sprinkle the tomatoes with the crumbs and drizzle lightly with the oil. Roast the tomatoes just until the crumbs are golden and the tomatoes are warmed through, about 8 minutes; you want them to hold their shape.

Serve hot, warm, or at room temperature.

Sicilian Potato Salad

There are so many veggies and fresh flavors in this dish that I almost hate to call it a potato salad, a name that conjures up visions of starchy, mayonnaise-y picnic plates. While this would certainly be great with grilled chicken at a backyard barbecue, the mix of colors and flavors make it equally compatible with all kinds of indoor fare. You could even fold in some leftover cooked protein, like salmon or sliced steak, to make it a one-dish meal.

Serves

4 TO 6

1 pound baby Yukon Gold potatoes

½ pound green beans, trimmed and cut into 1-inch pieces

⅓ cup extra-virgin olive oil

Grated zest of 1 lemon

¼ cup fresh lemon juice (one large lemon)

1 teaspoon dried Sicilian oregano

1 teaspoon kosher salt

½ small red onion, thinly sliced

1 cup cherry tomatoes, halved

½ cup pitted green olives, such as Castelvetrano or Cerignola

½ cup pitted black olives, such as kalamata

In a large saucepan, combine the potatoes with well-salted cold water to cover. Bring to a boil over high heat and continue to boil until the tip of a knife goes into the center of a potato with a little resistance, about 10 minutes. Add the green beans to the pot and cook for another 3 minutes.

While the potatoes boil, in a large bowl, whisk together the oil, lemon zest and juice, oregano, and ½ teaspoon of the salt. Place the sliced onion in a small bowl with cold water to cover.

Drain the potatoes and beans and when cool enough to handle, cut the potatoes in half. Add the potatoes to the dressing along with the beans. Drain the onion and add to the bowl along with the remaining ½ teaspoon salt, the tomatoes, and the green and black olives. Toss to coat everything with the dressing.

Serve warm or at room temperature.

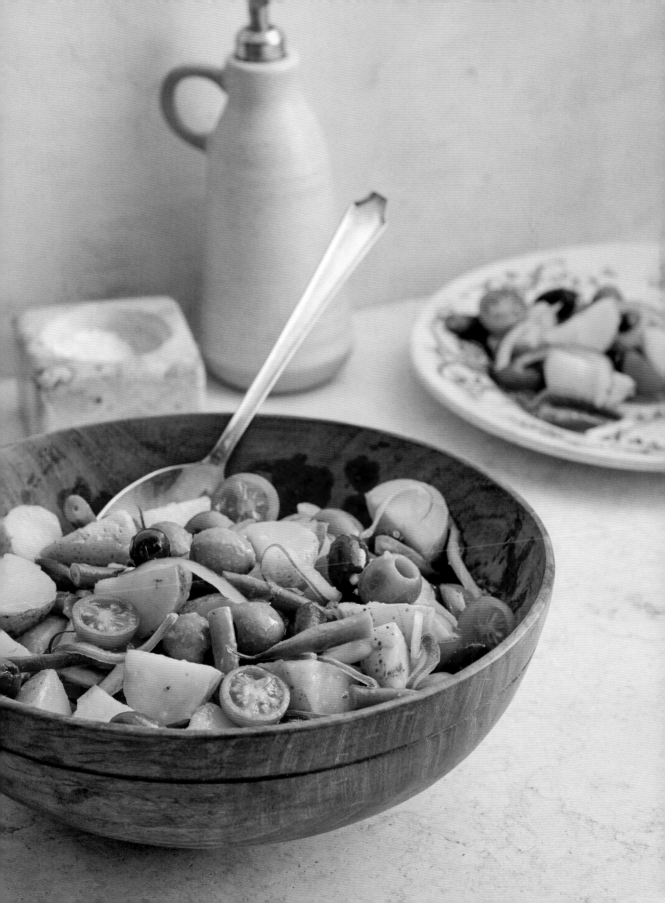

Spicy Lentils WITH Kale

Both as a side dish and as a building block for vegetarian meals like baked stuffed tomatoes or bell peppers, lentils are far and away my favorite kind of legume. I sometimes mix them with rice as the base of a protein-rich grain bowl, too. These aren't really spicy, the chiles just give them a little kick, but it is fine to leave them out entirely if you prefer. I use black or French Puy lentils because they hold their shape better, but if you only have regular green lentils, cook them just until tender.

Serves
6

◆

1¼ cups black lentils

½ small onion

3 garlic cloves

2 fresh thyme sprigs

1 fresh rosemary sprig

2 small dried Calabrian chiles
or ¼ teaspoon red pepper flakes

1 bay leaf

2 cups chopped lacinato
(Tuscan) kale

½ teaspoon kosher salt

In a saucepan, combine the lentils, onion, garlic, and 2 cups water and bring to a boil over high heat. When the water boils, reduce the heat to a simmer and add the thyme, rosemary, chiles, and bay leaf. Cook for 20 minutes.

Stir in the kale and cook until the lentils and kale are just tender, 5 to 10 minutes. Drain off any remaining water and discard the garlic, herb sprigs, chiles, and bay leaf. Season with the salt and serve.

Creamy Cannellini Beans

Think of this as the Italian equivalent of mashed potatoes, a smooth, creamy complement to any kind of meat or fish. As you cook down the beans, the liquid becomes silky and unctuous. Mash some or all of the beans as you prefer; I like to keep about half of them whole for a chunky texture.

Serves
4 TO 6

◆

2 (15-ounce) cans cannellini beans or 4 cups cooked beans (see below)

1 cup Parmesan Chicken Broth (page 64) or low-sodium store-bought chicken broth (see Hint)

3 or 4 garlic cloves, smashed and peeled

2 fresh rosemary sprigs

½ small lemon

1 teaspoon kosher salt

Best-quality extra-virgin olive oil, for drizzling

Drain off most of the liquid from the beans but do not rinse. Place the beans in a saucepan and use the chicken broth to rinse out any bean residue left in the can, adding it to the pot. Add the garlic, rosemary, lemon, and salt and bring to a simmer. Adjust the heat to keep the beans bubbling gently, partially cover, and cook until the cooking liquid has thickened a bit, stirring once or twice to keep the bottom from scorching, 20 to 25 minutes.

Remove the lemon and squeeze it into the pot, then discard the rind, rosemary, and garlic. Mash about half the beans to make a chunky, creamy mixture that still has some texture.

Serve the beans with a drizzle of your best olive oil.

HINT HINT ◆ If using plain chicken broth, add a piece of Parm rind to the pot to flavor the beans. Remove and discard the rind along with the other aromatics.

COOKING DRIED BEANS

Canned beans are a great convenience product and a staple in my pantry, but whenever I can, I love to use dried beans I've cooked myself. Not only are the flavor and texture generally superior, I can add flavorings to the cooking water, and the broth in the pot can be used in dishes as well. I don't even bother to soak them overnight—though if you do, you can deduct 10 minutes or so from the cooking time.

To cook dried beans from scratch, combine the beans in a pot with water to cover by at least 2 inches. Add a splash of olive oil, a clove or two of garlic, and a few sprigs of fresh herbs if you like. Bring to a boil, then immediately turn the heat to low and simmer until the beans are cooked through but not mushy, approximately 1 hour 15 minutes. Check your beans often and stir occasionally, making sure they remain covered with water; larger beans and older beans will take longer to cook. Store the cooked and cooled beans in some of their cooking liquid.

Warm Farro
WITH Mushrooms AND Brussels Sprouts

Grain salads are good keepers and filling enough to keep me going through a long afternoon. I think farro is especially nice for this kind of dish because it retains its nutty flavor and chewy texture so well. If you want to make this truly vegetarian—vegan, in fact—cook the farro in vegetable broth or water and omit the pancetta, and it will still be a completely satisfying and hearty dish. Be sure to have the sautéed veggies ready to go when the farro is finished cooking; the hot grain will absorb the flavorings better.

Serves

4

◆

1 cup pearled farro (see Hint)

2 cups Parmesan Chicken Broth (page 64) or low-sodium store-bought chicken or vegetable broth

2 garlic cloves, smashed and peeled

1 bay leaf

1½ teaspoons kosher salt

1 tablespoon extra-virgin olive oil

4 ounces diced pancetta

½ small red onion, diced

8 ounces cremini mushrooms, diced

8 ounces Brussels sprouts, trimmed and thinly sliced

2 tablespoons fresh lemon juice

½ cup salted roasted hazelnuts, chopped

¼ cup chopped fresh flat-leaf Italian parsley

In a medium saucepan, combine the farro, broth, garlic, bay leaf, and ½ teaspoon of the salt. Bring to a boil over medium-high heat, then reduce the heat to low, partially cover, and simmer until the farro is tender, about 15 minutes. Drain off any remaining cooking liquid, transfer the farro to a bowl, and fluff with a fork to separate the grain.

Meanwhile, in a large skillet, combine the oil and pancetta. Cook and stir over medium heat until the pancetta is browned and its fat has rendered, about 5 minutes. Use a slotted spoon to transfer the pancetta to a paper towel.

Add the onion, mushrooms, and ½ teaspoon salt to the same skillet and cook over medium heat, stirring often, until the mushrooms have released their liquid and are starting to brown, about 6 minutes.

Add the sprouts and stir until they are wilted and tender, 2 or 3 minutes. Season with the remaining ½ teaspoon salt and stir in the lemon juice.

Add the mushroom mixture to the bowl with the farro. Add the pancetta, nuts, and parsley and toss well to combine. Serve warm or at room temperature.

HINT HINT ◆ If your market doesn't carry pearled farro, which cooks more quickly than the semi-pearled or whole types, you can substitute either of the other two; just be aware you may need to cook the grain for as long as 40 minutes (for whole farro) and supplement the cooking liquid if the pan becomes too dry.

Grilled Artichokes

WITH GREEN OLIVE RELISH

Artichokes are always an unexpected yet welcome addition to a meal, and I find a few minutes on a hot grill (or grill pan) really takes their flavor to the next level. I serve this as a side at a barbecue, as a first course, or even part of an antipasto spread. You can parboil the artichokes up to 2 days in advance, then grill them just before serving. If the artichokes have been refrigerated, grill the rounded side for a few minutes first to warm through.

Serves

4

❖

2 large artichokes

2 garlic cloves,
smashed and peeled

2 bay leaves

Extra-virgin olive oil, for brushing

Green Olive Relish (page 55)

Break off and discard a row or two of the tough outer leaves from each artichoke. With a sharp knife, cut off the top ½ inch or so from each artichoke and trim off the stem. Stand the artichokes upright in a pot just large enough to hold them. Add the garlic, bay leaves, and enough water to come about one-third of the way up the sides of the artichokes.

Bring the water to a boil, then reduce the heat to medium-low and boil the artichokes until an outer leaf can be removed fairly easily (you don't want them falling off or the heart will be overcooked), 30 to 35 minutes. Place the artichokes upside down on a kitchen towel to drain.

Heat a ridged grill pan over high heat or prepare an outdoor grill. Halve the artichokes lengthwise through the stem end and use a small sharp knife to cut out the bristly choke, pulling out the spiky inner leaves along with the choke.

Brush the cut side of each artichoke half with oil and place cut side down on the grill or grill pan. Grill until nicely marked with grill lines, 4 to 5 minutes. Spoon a generous amount of the olive relish into the center of each artichoke half. Serve warm or at room temperature.

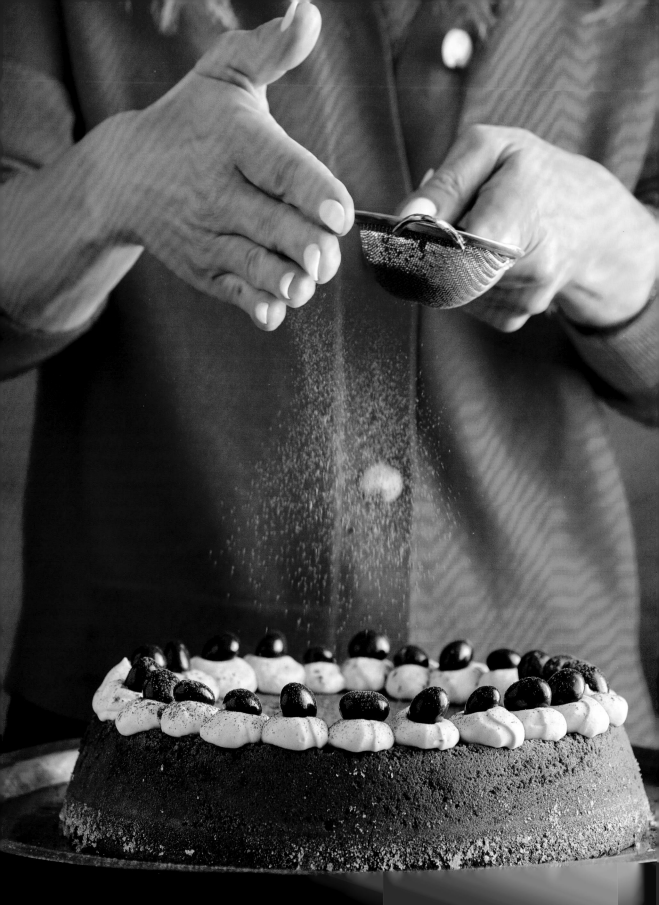

Nine

Dolce

Apulian Almond Cookies 246

Chocolate Orange Biscotti
with HAZELNUTS 247

Gingered Pumpkin Ricotta Cookies 250

Balsamic Chocolate Truffles 251

Bolognese Chocolate Torte
with COFFEE CREAM 252

Nonna Luna's Cherry Cake 255

Orange Olive Oil Cake
with APEROL GLAZE 257

Cannoli Rice Pudding 259

Basil Panna Cotta
with STRAWBERRIES 261

Plum Crostata 262

Lemon Affogato 265

Dessert

It completes the dining experience and ties it up with a bow. I'd even go so far as to say that ending meals on a sweet note may be *the* defining feature of La Dolce Vita, even if you are making an effort to eat more mindfully. I couldn't imagine entertaining without offering my guests a treat after dinner, and even when it's just my family, I always like to serve some kind of dessert. It doesn't have to be complicated, but there has be *something,* whether it's a piece of fruit, a cookie or two, or even just a bit of good chocolate.

It's certainly the way I grew up. My family didn't necessarily serve a fancy baked good or confection after dinner. We might just have put out some nuts in the shell, a bowl of tangerines, or some stone fruit in a bowl with ice water. Everyone would linger at the table, cracking nuts, using their knives to slice the fruit, sipping an espresso or glass of wine; it was a way to stretch out the meal and spend more time with the people we loved.

I'm not going to sugarcoat it (see what I did there?): The recipes in this chapter are not *quite* as nutritionally dense or as health supporting as some of the others in this book, and that's okay. They are not trying to be! But they *are* designed to pack a flavorful punch in every bite; their concentrated flavors mean you feel treated without eating a lot. And even though I can't in good conscience say they are "healthy," just about all of them incorporate one or more of my superfoods, whether it's a nut, fruit, or fresh herb.

If you are looking for cooks who have figured out how to make great-tasting desserts without refined sugar or flour or dairy, there are plenty of them out there producing treats that will at least appease your sweet tooth. I'm just not that cook and never will be. If I can't have the real thing, I'd rather have fruit than something made with fake sugar or some kind of ingredient swap.

If you are worried about having sweets around, do as I do and bake when you plan to have family over; if there are leftovers, pack them up and send them home with your guests. If you are making cookies, just bake as many as you need for the occasion at hand and freeze the rest of the dough to bake off at a later date.

Apulian Almond Cookies

One afternoon in Puglia, I stopped in to a café for a coffee shakerato and they served a few of these cookies along with my drink. It was love at first bite! It took me a minute to re-create the crunchy-chewy texture, but I think I nailed it. If you are an impatient baker, you have just found your ideal cookie. You don't need to wait for butter to soften—in fact this recipe is dairy- *and* gluten-free—or let the dough rest, so these can be in the oven about 10 minutes after you start the recipe. And if you are in the habit of keeping almond flour on hand, it's also a convenient pantry recipe. I like them flavored with honey, as they would be made in Italy, but you can substitute the same amount of maple syrup or even agave. This recipe halves easily, but they are good keepers, so go for a whole batch!

Makes

ABOUT 36 COOKIES

2 large eggs

4 cups almond flour

½ cup (packed) light brown sugar

¼ cup mild-flavored honey (such as thyme or clover)

½ teaspoon kosher salt

½ cup granulated sugar

36 whole almonds

Preheat the oven to 325°F. Line two sheet pans with parchment paper.

In a large bowl, beat the eggs until uniformly colored. Add the flour, brown sugar, honey, and salt and stir with a rubber spatula until completely combined into a moist dough, 2 or 3 minutes. The dough will have the look and consistency of light brown sugar.

Place the granulated sugar in a small bowl. Scoop the dough by tablespoons and roll each scoop into a football shape. Roll the cookies in the sugar and place on the prepared baking sheets, leaving 1 inch between them. Press 1 almond deep into the top of each cookie to flatten them slightly.

Place the two sheet pans on different oven racks. Bake the cookies for 9 to 10 minutes, then switch the positions of the pans and continue to bake until just turning golden brown on top, 17 to 19 minutes in total. Don't worry if they crack; that is perfectly fine. Without removing the sheet pans, turn off the oven and let the cookies dry out for another 10 minutes.

Cool completely on the pans, then store in an airtight container for up to 5 days.

Chocolate Orange Biscotti

WITH HAZELNUTS

One of the nicest things about biscotti is how easy it is to change the flavorings, depending on what's on your shelf and what combos spark your creativity on any given day. Here I've used a time-honored combination—chocolate and orange—plus hazelnuts for richness and crunch. Italy is justly proud of its hazelnuts, with the very best coming from the Piedmont region, and they are the biscotti baker's nut of choice. I like to use salted roasted nuts, but if you can only find raw hazelnuts, up the salt to ½ teaspoon and give the nuts a quick toast (see Hint) before chopping them to get a similar result.

Makes
ABOUT 24 BISCOTTI

8 tablespoons (1 stick) unsalted butter, at room temperature

¾ cup sugar

2 teaspoons grated orange zest

¼ teaspoon kosher salt

2 large eggs

2 cups all-purpose flour

1½ teaspoons baking powder

1½ cups semisweet or bittersweet chocolate chunks

⅓ cup chopped salted roasted hazelnuts

¼ cup diced candied orange peel

HINT HINT ◆ Toast hazelnuts on a sheet pan in a 350°F oven until they smell nutty, about 10 minutes. Let them cool for 15 minutes before chopping.

Preheat the oven to 350°F. Line a baking sheet with parchment paper.

In a stand mixer, combine the butter, sugar, orange zest, and salt. Beat on medium speed until light, about 1 minute. Add the eggs, 1 at a time, beating until each is incorporated. Add the flour and baking powder and beat until nearly incorporated. Remove the bowl from the mixer and add ½ cup of the chocolate chunks, the nuts, and the candied orange peel, stirring by hand with a rubber spatula until the last bits of flour and the add-ins are incorporated.

Form the dough into a 12-inch log about 3 inches in diameter and place on the prepared baking sheet. Bake until the log is light golden brown, about 40 minutes. Remove the baking sheet from the oven but don't turn off the oven. Let the log cool on the baking sheet for 30 minutes.

Carefully transfer the dough log to a cutting board. Using a serrated knife, slice the log on the diagonal to make long slices about ½ inch thick. Arrange the slices on the same baking sheet, cut sides down, and return them to the oven. Bake until the cut surfaces are lightly golden, about 15 minutes. Transfer the biscotti to a rack to cool completely.

Place the remaining 1 cup chocolate chunks in a glass measuring cup and melt in the microwave on high, heating in 20-second intervals and stirring after each. Dip the biscotti in the melted chocolate, coating about one-third of each. Return to the rack to allow the chocolate to set, about 30 minutes. Store the biscotti in an airtight container for up to 1 week.

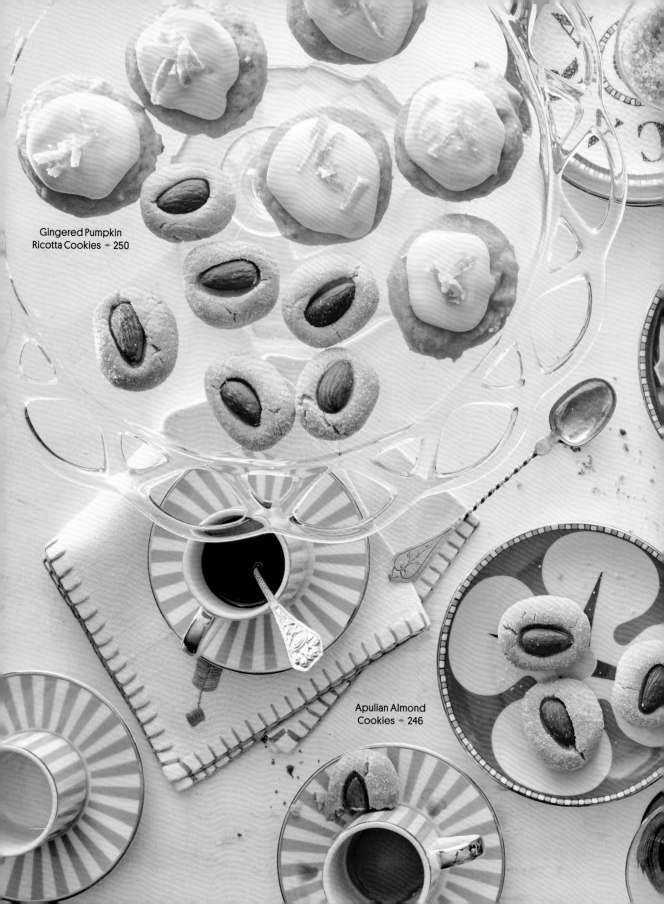

Gingered Pumpkin
Ricotta Cookies → 250

Apulian Almond
Cookies → 246

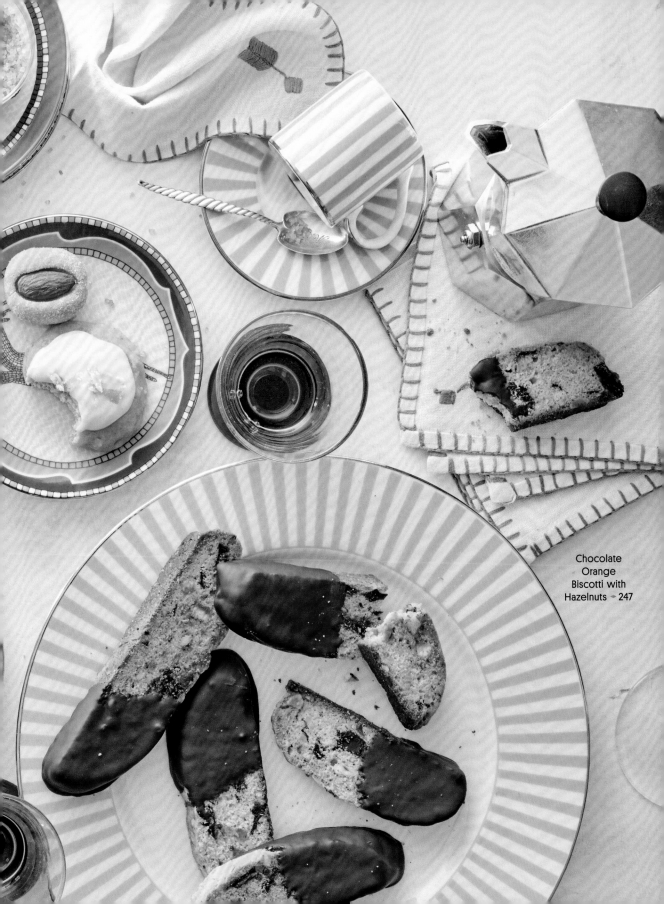

Chocolate
Orange
Biscotti with
Hazelnuts ⟶ 247

Gingered Pumpkin Ricotta Cookies

My grandmother's beloved lemon ricotta cookies are hard to improve upon, but I thought it might be fun to give them a fall spin and sneak a little bit of beta-carotene-rich pumpkin in there! I love how light and bouncy these are, almost more like a little tea cake than a cookie. Pumpkin and maple are a classic fall combo and here they give an Italian favorite more of an American sensibility. Like all the cookies in this chapter, these are not terribly sweet, but they have a nice snap from both ground and candied ginger. Ginger has healing properties, so enjoy the cookie with a cup of ginger tea if you have a troubled tummy.

Makes
ABOUT 36 COOKIES

❖

FOR THE COOKIES

2½ cups all-purpose flour

1 teaspoon baking powder

¾ teaspoon ground cinnamon

1½ teaspoons ground ginger

1 teaspoon kosher salt

8 tablespoons (1 stick) unsalted butter, at room temperature

1 cup granulated sugar

1 cup (packed) light brown sugar

2 large eggs

1 cup whole-milk ricotta cheese

½ cup canned pumpkin puree

FOR THE ICING

1½ cups confectioners' sugar

5 to 6 tablespoons pure maple syrup

Pinch of kosher salt

¼ cup candied ginger, cut in thin slivers

Preheat the oven to 375°F. Line two sheet pans with parchment paper.

Make the cookies: In a medium bowl, combine the flour, baking powder, cinnamon, ginger, and salt. Set aside.

In a stand mixer, combine the butter, granulated sugar, and brown sugar and beat on medium-high speed until light and fluffy, about 3 minutes. Add the eggs, 1 at a time, beating until incorporated, scraping down the sides of the bowl after each addition. Add the ricotta and pumpkin and beat to combine. Add the flour mixture and beat on low speed until just incorporated.

Use a 2-tablespoon cookie scoop to portion the dough on the prepared baking sheets, allowing at least an inch between them.

Bake one sheet until the cookies become lightly golden at the edges, 13 to 15 minutes. Repeat with the second sheet. Let the cookies cool on the sheet pan for 20 minutes, then transfer to a wire rack to cool completely.

Meanwhile, make the icing: In a small bowl, combine the confectioners' sugar, 4 tablespoons of the maple syrup, and the salt and stir until smooth. The icing should be very thick, but if it is not spoonable, add more maple syrup as needed. Spoon about 1 teaspoon of the icing on each cooled cookie and use the back of the spoon to spread it to the edges. Place a few pieces of ginger on each cookie. Let the icing set until dry to the touch, then store the cookies in an airtight container. These are best eaten within a day or two of baking.

Balsamic Chocolate Truffles

It's amazing what you can do with just a handful of ingredients, especially if you opt for better quality. If you have been saving a mellow, aged balsamic for a special occasion, that day has come. The vinegar's fruity, soft tones blend deliciously with chocolate here. If you don't have aged balsamic, reduce the balsamic you have on hand over low heat by about half to give it a bit more body and less bite. You don't need to use the deepest, darkest chocolate for these; something in the 60% to 65% cacao range does the trick nicely. I make these quite small—just a teaspoon each—because they are *that* rich.

Makes
24 SMALL TRUFFLES

8 ounces bittersweet chocolate, preferably in bar form, coarsely chopped

¼ cup heavy cream

2 tablespoons aged balsamic vinegar

1 cup unsweetened cocoa powder

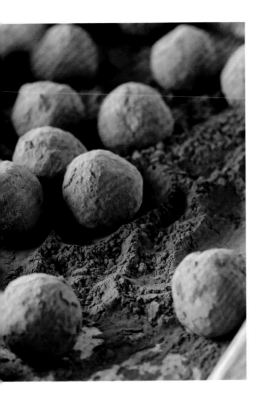

In a small microwave-safe bowl, combine the chocolate and cream and microwave on high for 40 seconds. Stir with a silicone spatula for 5 seconds, then return to the microwave and continue to heat in 20-second intervals until the chocolate is almost entirely melted, about 1 minute 20 seconds total. Stir until completely smooth, then stir in the vinegar until thoroughly combined. Cover the bowl and refrigerate for 1 hour or until fairly firm.

Cover a plate with a piece of parchment and place the cocoa powder in a shallow bowl. One at a time, scoop up a heaping teaspoonful of the chocolate mixture and use your hands to roll it into a ball about the size of a small cherry. Drop each ball in the cocoa powder as you finish shaping it, turning it to coat completely, then set it on the parchment-lined plate.

Store the truffles in the refrigerator in a covered container for a week or longer—if you can resist eating them all!

Bolognese Chocolate Torte

WITH COFFEE CREAM

This elegant dessert ticks so many boxes: It's gluten-free, can be made ahead of time, and is not too sweet. And unlike its cousin, the Neapolitan torta Caprese, it doesn't contain nuts or nut flour—all of which make it a good choice for entertaining. Best of all, it couldn't be easier to make. The only trick is taking care not to overbake it; better to have the very center a tad soft than to allow the exterior of the cake to become dry. In Italy, you would find this served with a simple dusting of confectioners' sugar, but I like to dress it up with a coffee-flavored whipped cream stabilized with a bit of mascarpone.

Serves
8 TO 10

FOR THE CAKE

Softened butter and sugar
for the pan

8 ounces bittersweet chocolate,
roughly chopped

8 tablespoons (1 stick) unsalted
butter, diced

5 large eggs, separated

1 teaspoon espresso powder

1 cup granulated sugar

¼ cup potato starch

½ teaspoon kosher salt

FOR THE COFFEE CREAM

½ cup cold heavy cream

1 teaspoon espresso powder

¼ cup mascarpone cheese

2 teaspoons confectioners' sugar

Chocolate-covered espresso
beans, for garnish

Make the cake: Preheat the oven to 350°F. Butter a 9-inch round baking pan and line the bottom with a round of parchment paper. Butter the paper. Dust the pan with some sugar, turning to coat all the surfaces, then tap out the excess.

In a glass measuring cup, combine the chocolate and butter and microwave on high in 30-second intervals, stirring well after each interval and stopping when there are still a few bits of unmelted chocolate visible. Stir until smooth, then set aside to cool slightly.

In a stand mixer, combine the egg yolks, espresso powder, and the granulated sugar and beat on medium speed until the mixture is thick, fluffy, and pale, about 2 minutes. In a separate bowl, beat the egg whites until stiff peaks form, about 2 minutes.

Add the cooled chocolate to the egg yolk mixture and beat on low to combine. Add the potato starch and salt and beat again until just combined. Remove the bowl from the mixer stand. In three batches, fold the whipped whites into the chocolate mixture with a rubber spatula, taking care not to deflate the whites. Pour the batter into the prepared pan.

Bake until the top is set and a toothpick inserted in the center comes out with moist crumbs attached, 32 to 35 minutes. Be careful not to overbake.

Run a sharp knife around the edges of the cake, then set the pan on a wire rack to cool completely.

Make the coffee cream: In the bowl of a stand mixer, combine the cream and espresso powder and stir by hand until it dissolves. Snap on the whisk, add the mascarpone and confectioners' sugar, and beat on high until stiff peaks form.

To serve, carefully invert the cake onto a large plate. Pipe rosettes of the whipped cream onto the cake and decorate with the espresso beans.

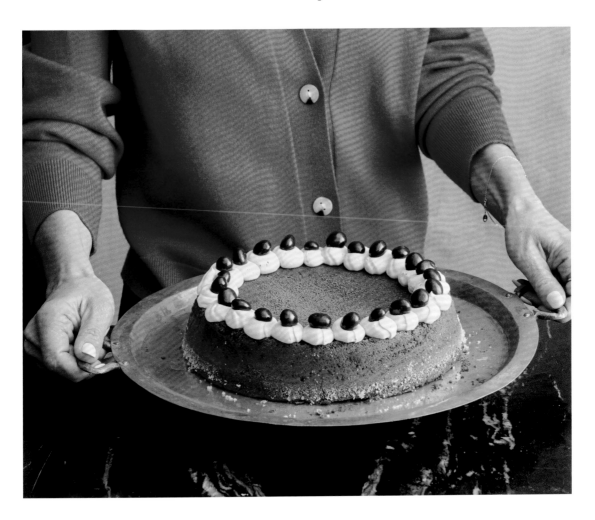

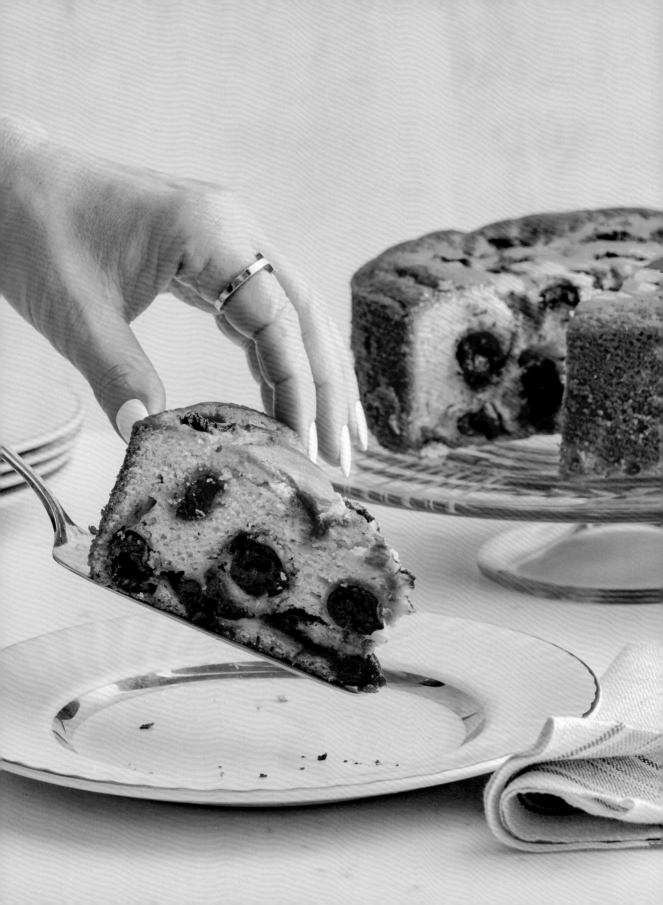

Nonna Luna's Cherry Cake

Developing this cake was a special request from my aunt Raffy, who remembered her mother making it when she was young. I wanted to bring back all those sweet memories for her, and she said I hit the mark with this. Made with frozen cherries, this is an anytime cake, but it's especially luscious made with fresh cherries. If using frozen, don't thaw them; use them straight from the freezer, brushing off any ice crystals or bits of frozen juice before adding them to the batter.

Serves
8 TO 10

◆

8 tablespoons (1 stick) unsalted butter, at room temperature

1 cup granulated sugar

1 cup plain whole-milk Greek yogurt, at room temperature

3 large eggs, at room temperature

¾ teaspoon pure vanilla extract

¼ teaspoon almond extract

1¾ cups all-purpose flour

2 teaspoons baking powder

½ teaspoon kosher salt

1 (10- to 12-ounce) bag frozen cherries or 10 to 12 ounces pitted fresh cherries

2 tablespoons turbinado sugar

Amarena cherries (optional), for topping

Preheat the oven to 350°F. Spritz the bottom and sides of an 8-inch round cake pan with cooking spray and line the bottom with a round of parchment paper.

In a stand mixer, beat together the butter and granulated sugar on medium speed until light and fluffy, about 3 minutes. Beat in the yogurt and 2 tablespoons water and mix on medium, scraping the sides once or twice until fully incorporated. Reduce the speed to low and add the eggs, 1 at a time, making sure each is fully incorporated before adding the next. Beat in the vanilla and almond extracts.

In a medium bowl, whisk together the flour, baking powder, and salt. Add the dry ingredients to the batter and mix on low speed until almost combined. Set aside 8 to 10 of the cherries and add the rest to the batter, using a rubber spatula to fold them in by hand and to incorporate any final bits of flour.

Scrape the batter into the prepared cake pan, smoothing the top. Slice the reserved cherries in half and arrange them decoratively on the surface of the cake, cut sides down. Sprinkle with the turbinado sugar.

Bake until a toothpick inserted in the center comes out almost clean, the top is golden brown, and the cake has pulled away from the sides of the pan, 1 hour 5 minutes to 1 hour 10 minutes.

Let the cake cool in the pan on a wire rack for at least 30 minutes. If desired, serve the cake topped with Amarena cherries and some syrup from the jar.

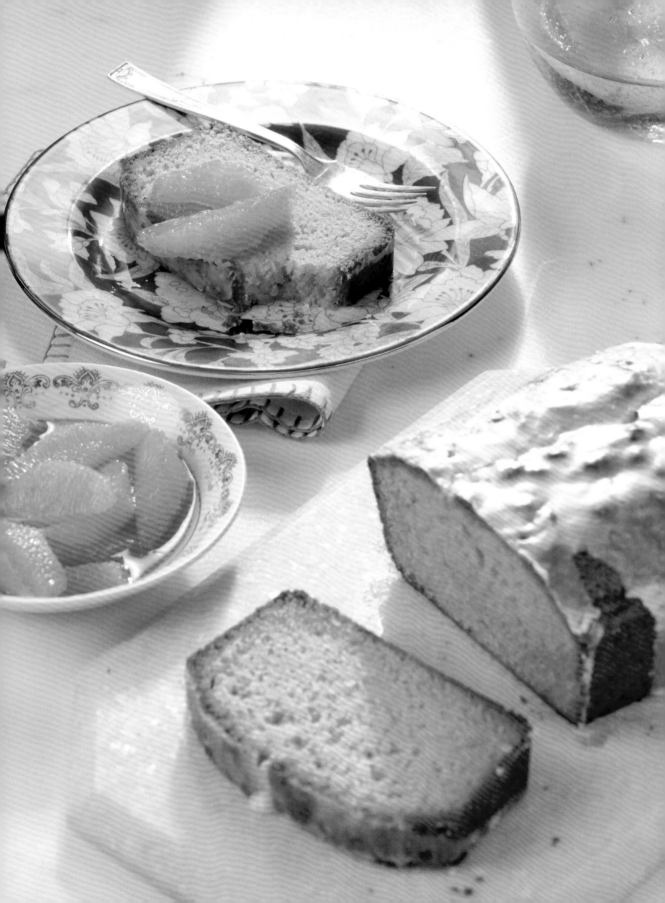

Orange Olive Oil Cake

WITH APEROL GLAZE

The best citrus in Italy comes from the Amalfi Coast and specifically Sorrento. They use their abundant citrus harvest to flavor all sorts of things, including olive oil, and an orange-flavored oil originally inspired this cake. Flavored oils are not as easy to come by in the United States, so I have adapted the recipe to use the juice and zest of oranges instead, and it is just as fragrant and delicious. Aperol in the glaze adds a little digestivo action.

Serves

8

1 cup granulated sugar

2 oranges

3 large eggs, at room temperature

¼ cup whole milk, at room temperature

¾ cup extra-virgin olive oil

1½ cups all-purpose flour

2 teaspoons baking powder

½ teaspoon kosher salt

2 tablespoons Aperol

1½ cups confectioners' sugar

Preheat the oven to 350°F. Spritz a 9 × 5-inch loaf pan with cooking spray. Line the pan with a piece of parchment paper, allowing the excess to overhang the long sides.

Place the granulated sugar in the bowl of a stand mixer. Zest the oranges on a Microplane directly over the bowl. (Reserve the zested oranges for serving.) Use your fingertips to work the zest into the sugar until it is fragrant and pale orange. With the mixer on medium-low, add the eggs, 1 at a time, and beat until fluffy. Beat in the milk and then gradually beat in the oil until fully incorporated.

In a medium bowl, whisk together the flour, baking powder, and salt to blend. Add the flour mixture to the batter and beat on low speed until nearly combined, giving it a few final strokes by hand with a rubber spatula to incorporate the last bits of flour.

Spread the batter in the prepared pan and tap the pan on the countertop once or twice to release any air pockets.

Bake until the top bounces back when pressed with your fingertip and a toothpick inserted in the center of the cake comes out with a few moist crumbs attached, 35 to 40 minutes.

Let the cake cool in the pan on a wire rack for 15 minutes. Remove the cake from the pan to the rack to cool completely.

CONTINUES

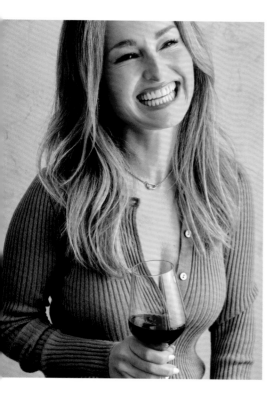

To serve, use a sharp knife to slice off all the white pith from the zested oranges. Working over a bowl to catch the juice, cut down each side of the membranes to free the orange segments, letting the segments drop into the bowl. Toss with the Aperol.

Sift the confectioners' sugar into a medium bowl and add 2 tablespoons of juice from the bowl of orange segments. Stir to make a thick but pourable glaze, adding a bit more juice if needed.

Drizzle the glaze over the completely cooled loaf, allowing it to run down the sides. Let the glaze set until hardened.

Cut into slices and serve topped with a few orange segments and their juices.

Cannoli Rice Pudding

Rice pudding may seem like a classic British nursery dessert, but it is popular in Italy, where it is often served topped with sprinkles at the holidays. Adding some ricotta to the mixture is a nod to the yummy filling you find in cannoli, but here you get all the creamy sweetness without the hassle of frying the shells. A handful of mini chocolate chips in the pudding and a sprinkle of pistachios on top completes the picture and adds some welcome texture. Don't stir the chips into the pudding if it's even slightly warm, as they will melt and leave streaks in the pudding.

Serves

6

◆

3 cups whole milk,
plus more as needed

¼ cup Arborio or other
short-grain rice

½ teaspoon pure vanilla extract

¼ teaspoon kosher salt

¼ cup whole-milk ricotta cheese

⅓ cup mini chocolate chips

1 tablespoon unsweetened cocoa
powder, for dusting

5 or 6 salted roasted pistachios,
very finely chopped or grated

In a saucepan, combine the milk, rice, vanilla, and salt and bring to a simmer over medium heat. Reduce the heat to very low and cook, stirring every 5 to 10 minutes, until the rice is very tender and the pudding is thick and creamy, about 50 minutes. If the rice is still a bit al dente, cook for another 10 to 15 minutes, adding a bit more milk if the mixture gets too thick.

Meanwhile, use an immersion blender or small blender to whip the ricotta until light and smooth.

When the pudding is done, stir the ricotta into the pudding and refrigerate until cold, at least 1 hour.

To serve, stir in the chocolate chips. Scoop the pudding into coupe glasses or small dishes. Place the cocoa powder in a small sieve and tap lightly over each serving to dust the top. Sprinkle the pistachios on one side of each portion.

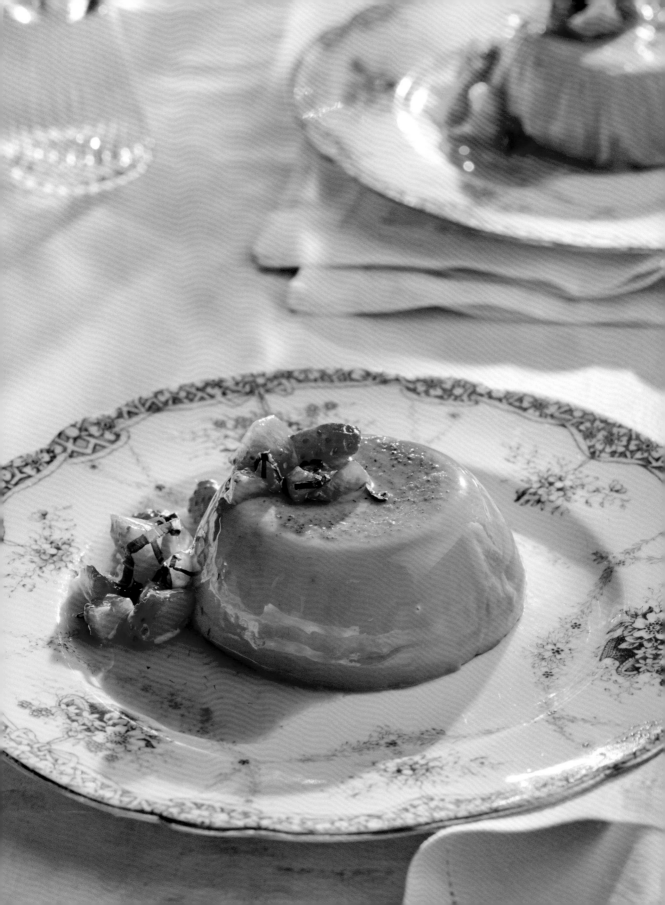

Basil Panna Cotta

WITH STRAWBERRIES

These creamy puddings are a go-to dessert for entertaining throughout Italy because they can be made ahead of time and are easy to dress up. Even with all that going for it, panna cotta is kind of bland to me, and usually the last thing that catches my eye on a menu. But I know I'm in the minority here—panna cotta is a top seller at my restaurants—so I wanted to see if I could make a panna cotta I really enjoyed, and this one fits that bill perfectly. It always surprises people with its chic green color and subtle herbaceous flavor. It's nicest in summer when both berries and basil are at their most flavorful.

Serves
6

1 cup whole milk

1 cup heavy cream

½ cup (loosely packed) fresh basil leaves

2 teaspoons unflavored gelatin

½ cup sugar

Generous pinch of kosher salt

FOR SERVING

1 pint strawberries, cut into small cubes or sliced

1 tablespoon sugar

Tiny pinch of kosher salt

6 fresh basil or mint leaves, slivered

In a blender, combine the milk, cream, and basil and blitz for a few seconds to chop the basil. Pour into a small saucepan and bring to a simmer over medium heat. Remove from the heat and let stand for 15 minutes to infuse the milk mixture with the basil.

In a small bowl, mix the gelatin with 2 tablespoons water and set aside for 5 minutes.

Strain the basil-infused milk into a bowl, discarding the basil, then return the milk to the saucepan. Add the sugar, salt, and softened gelatin and bring to a simmer over medium heat. Stir for a minute or two to dissolve the sugar.

Divide the mixture among six small ramekins (5 to 6 ounces) or custard cups (they will not be completely filled). Chill until firm, at least 4 hours and preferably overnight.

To serve, place the strawberries in a medium bowl and sprinkle with the sugar and salt. Stir to combine and let the berries macerate for 20 minutes or so to release their juices. Stir in the basil.

To serve, run a small knife around the edges of each ramekin and dip the ramekin briefly into a bowl of hot water to loosen it. Invert the panna cottas onto individual dessert plates and spoon some of the berries and their juices onto each serving.

Plum Crostata

Crostatas are very popular in Italy and not only do we eat them after dinner, but any leftovers get served the next day for breakfast! They are a great way to use up fruit that might be on its way out. My mother even filled them with jam when she didn't have any fresh fruit. Because they're free-form, I find them a lot less stressful to make than pies. They don't need to be baked as long, either, because there is much less filling, and they also don't need to cool completely before serving. [Remind me why anyone makes pies?] Spreading a bit of flour on the crust is a trick I picked up from cookbook author Susan Spungen, and it really helps keep the juices from running onto the baking sheet.

Serves
6

FOR THE CRUST

10 tablespoons [1¼ sticks] very cold unsalted butter, cut into ½-inch pieces

1½ cups all-purpose flour, plus more for rolling the dough

2 tablespoons sugar

½ teaspoon kosher salt

3 tablespoons ice water, plus more if needed

FOR THE FILLING

2 tablespoons all-purpose flour

4 to 6 tablespoons granulated sugar, depending on the sweetness of your fruit

4 red or black plums, halved, pitted, and cut in ¼-inch slices

2 tablespoons heavy cream or whole milk

¼ cup sliced almonds

2 tablespoons turbinado sugar or additional granulated sugar

Make the crust: In a food processor, combine the butter, flour, sugar, and salt and pulse on and off until the mixture resembles coarse meal. Add the ice water and pulse until it begins to form clumps.

Turn the dough onto a sheet of plastic wrap and press the clumps together to form a rough, thick disk. (It's okay if there are just a few dry bits; if it seems very dry, sprinkle with a bit more ice water.) Wrap tightly in the plastic and refrigerate for at least 1 hour and up to 2 days.

Preheat the oven to 400°F. Line a baking sheet with parchment paper.

On a lightly floured surface, roll the pastry dough into an oval shape about 18 inches long, dusting the surface with flour and flipping the dough every 3 or 4 passes of the rolling pin to keep it from sticking. Roll the dough onto your rolling pin, then unroll onto the center of the prepared baking sheet.

Sprinkle the flour onto the pastry and with your fingers spread to within an inch of the edges. Sprinkle the granulated sugar over the flour. Mound the plums on the pastry, spreading them to within about 2 inches of the edges, then use the parchment paper to help fold the pastry up and over the filling, pleating as you go. Brush the folded edge of the crust with the cream and sprinkle both the crust and the plums with the sliced almonds and turbinado sugar.

Bake until the crust is deep golden brown and the fruit juices are bubbling, 35 to 40 minutes. Serve warm or at room temperature.

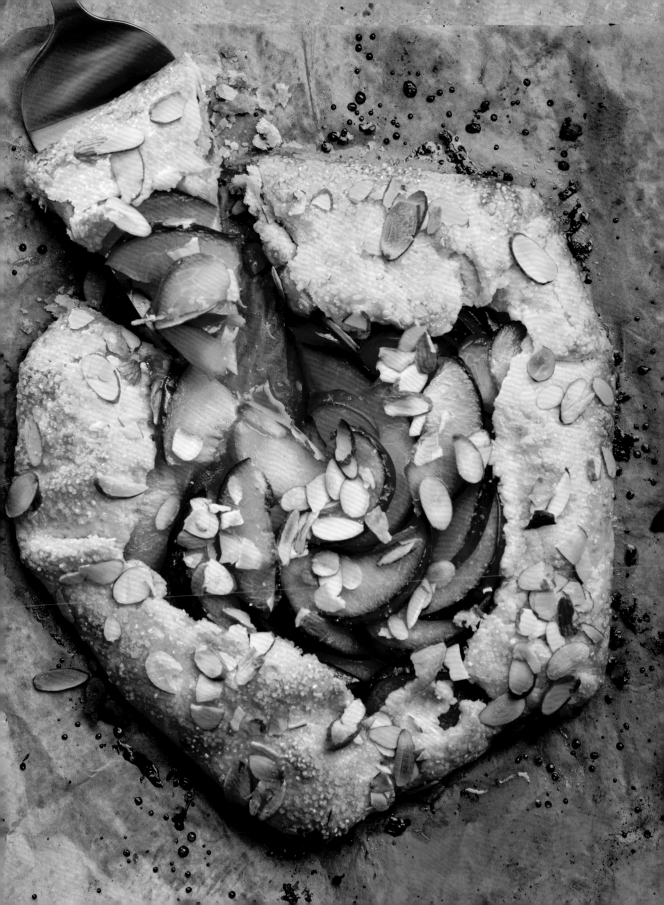

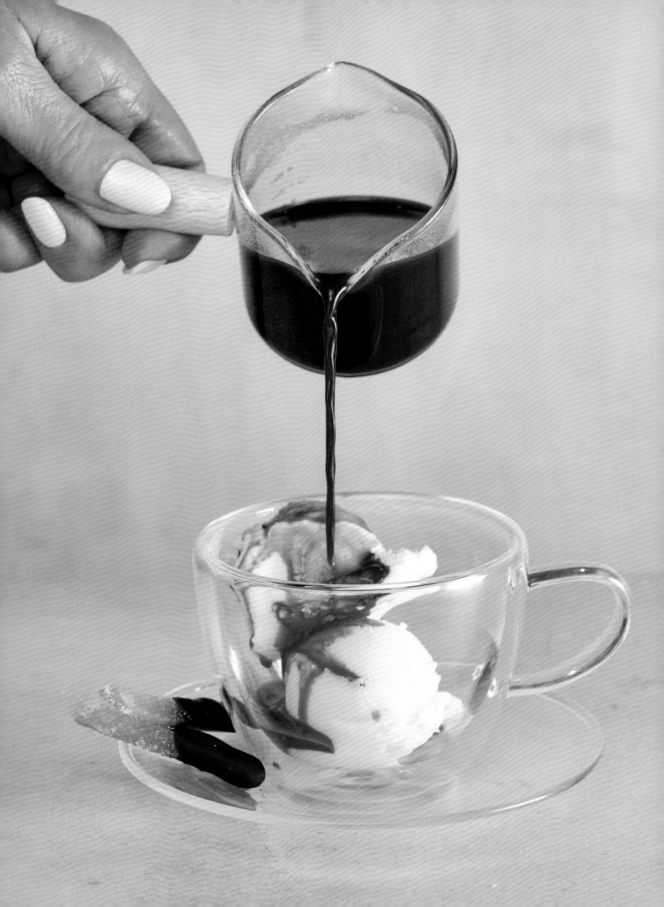

Lemon Affogato

My family served affogato a lot when I was growing up, especially in the summer as a way to cool down the espresso that is always served at the end of a meal. For the kids of course it was more gelato than espresso, but we always got a little drizzle over our serving, and it made us feel very grown-up! We used vanilla gelato, but I figured it might be even more delicious with lemon—after all, espresso is always served with a lemon twist—plus, I could never have a cookbook without at least one lemon dessert. That just wouldn't be right! The candied peel dials up the lemon even further, but if you want to skip those steps, this qualifies as a no-cook, no-sweat dessert you can bust out anytime.

Serves

4

1 lemon

¾ cup sugar, plus more for rolling the lemon strips

2 ounces bittersweet chocolate, chopped

1 pint lemon gelato

4 shots (about ¼ cup each) freshly brewed espresso

To make the candied lemon peel, use a sharp paring knife to slice off the lemon rind (including the white pith) in long strips. Cut the strips into narrow pieces about ¼ inch wide. Squeeze the juice of the lemon into a small bowl and set aside.

Place the rind in a small saucepan with water to cover and bring to a boil over high heat. When the water boils, drain the lemon strips, then return them to the pot with fresh water. Bring to a boil again and drain again.

Add the sugar, lemon juice, and 1 cup fresh water to the saucepan and bring to a boil. Add the lemon strips and boil, without stirring, until the pith is translucent, about 30 minutes.

Meanwhile, spread some sugar on a plate. Set a wire rack on a sheet pan.

Use a slotted spoon to remove the lemon strips to the sugar-covered plate and roll the strips to coat in the sugar. Set the sugared rinds on the wire rack to dry overnight. (You can save the lemon syrup for cocktails or another use!)

Place two-thirds of the chocolate in a small coffee mug. Place the mug in a saucepan with an inch of simmering water and heat until the chocolate melts. Stir in the remaining chopped chocolate, stirring until smooth. Dip the sugared rinds into the chocolate, coating them about halfway, and place on a sheet of parchment to harden.

To serve, place two small scoops of the gelato in serving dishes or heatproof glasses. Pour a shot of hot espresso over each serving and decorate with a strip or two of candied peel. Serve immediately!

Acknowledgments

As always, I am grateful to the extended team of individuals whose talents have contributed to this book.

At Rodale, my publishing team, led by publisher Diana Baroni and executive editor Dervla Kelly, aided by Katherine Leak, encouraged me to deepen my exploration of the healthy side of Italian cooking (shout-out, too, to Raquel Pelzel for early guidance in the process); art director Jenny Davis oversaw the good-looking design, and Richard Elman, Kate Slate, and Loren Noveck provided essential production support. Thanks also to Odette Fleming, Kelly Doyle, and the rest of the marketing and PR folks who helped connect my book with readers.

To create the photographs that truly bring a cookbook to life, I was lucky enough to work with the divine Ray Kachatorian, whose perpetual good humor and love of food make the long days of shooting pure pleasure. J. Horton (lighting director); Jen Barguiarena (props); Sophie Clark (food stylist); and culinary assistants David Boyle, Alyssa Montes Garcia, and Elle Debel all made sure every dish looked as delicious as it tasted.

Behind the scenes, Suzanne Gluck, Eric Greenspan, Mary Grace Detmer, Natasha Wynnyk, and Pam Krauss provided key support to make this project possible.

And of course, no book could happen without the encouragement of my trusted tasting panel, cheerleading squad, and partners in crime, Jade Thompson and Shane Farley. They are my reasons for cooking every day and staying healthy the Super-Italian way!

Index